Ethics Handbook for Energy Healing Practitioners

Ethics Handbook for Energy Healing Practitioners

A Guide for the Professional Practice of
Energy Medicine and Energy Psychology

David Feinstein, PhD
with Donna Eden

Energy Psychology Press

Petaluma, CA 95953

www.energypsychologypress.com

Library of Congress Cataloging-in-Publication Data

Feinstein, David.
Ethics handbook for energy healing practitioners : a guide for the professional practice of energy medicine and energy psychology / David Feinstein ; with Donna Eden. -- 2nd.
     p. ; cm.
   Includes bibliographical references.
   ISBN 978-1-60415-290-6 (hardcover)
   1. Energy medicine--Moral and ethical aspects. I. Eden, Donna. II. Title.
   [DNLM: 1. Therapeutic Touch--ethics. 2. Professional-Patient Relations-
-ethics. WB 890]
   RZ421.F45 2011
   615.8'51--dc22
                                     2011009772
                            © 2011, 2024 David Feinstein

Typeset in Minion Pro
Printed in USA
Second Edition

10 9 8 7 6 5 4 3 2 1

Contents

Acknowledgments

A document of this nature builds upon the wisdom garnered by innumerable health-care practitioners throughout history and by those they have tended. Ethical guidelines are a profession's evolving legacy, guiding its members in how to serve the public at the highest standard possible.

Ethics statements used by the Acupuncture and Oriental Medicine Alliance, the American Holistic Nurses Association, the American Psychological Association (APA), the Association for Comprehensive Energy Psychology (ACEP), the Barbara Brennan School of Healing, the British Complementary Medicine Association, the Council on Healing, the Energy Kinesiology Association, the Somatic Therapist Association, and the Therapeutic Massage and Bodywork Board were all consulted and had influence in the development of this document. The collective thinking these professions have devoted to their aspirations and ethical standards is the bedrock of this document and gratefully acknowledged.

Initial ideas on how to approach some of the ethical vignettes in this handbook were formulated by a team of energy medicine practitioners trained by Donna Eden and chaired by Debra Hurt Burchard. Members of that team included Francie Boyce, Helen Campbell, Marjorie Fein, Ellen Ferguson, Jan Firstenberg, Sue Gridley, Donna Kemper, Tammy Komp, Sue Powell, June Scott, and Janel Volk-Hubbard. We are indebted to these individuals for their strong contributions to the discussion of ethical vignettes. Carolyn Schuyler read an almost-final draft of the book and added a number of topics that have made this a more comprehensive treatment of ethical issues for energy healing practitioners.

Editorial assistance from Connie Kosmann, Jennifer Massey, Ellen Meredith, and Lily Splane is gratefully acknowledged.

Quotations from *The Educated Heart* (2nd ed., 2005) by Nina McIntosh are placed throughout the chapter on "Ethical Dilemmas You May Face," with permission from the publisher, Lippincott Williams & Wilkins.

Disclaimer: This Handbook is educational in nature and is provided for instructional purposes, not as legal advice. Ethics laws and regulations differ among countries and regions, professional organizations, and subdisciplines. Even the term "Energy Healer," used throughout this book, cannot be used by unlicensed practitioners in certain states, yet "Energy Healing Practitioner" can be. This illustrates the importance of knowing your local, as well as national, laws and regulations. Please consult an attorney or a member of your professional organization for counsel on specific ethical dilemmas.

Introduction

When we started the two-year Eden Energy Medicine Certification Program in 2005, our students ranged from physicians and other seasoned health-care professionals to those who had never had a course in ethics. We developed a case study approach to teaching ethics, which proved highly engaging for our 220 students of all levels of experience. The human dilemmas in ethical issues cut across all bounds, and our role-plays, mock ethics hearings, and penetrating discussions of the core issues were illuminating for us as instructors as well as for the students. We have tried to capture this interactive case study approach in this book as well.

We quickly make it clear to our students that ethics are far more than a list of rules that will restrict them or requirements that should put fear in their hearts. Ethics are the principles adopted by practitioners within a field to translate the *desire to serve* into the profession's evolving wisdom about *how best to serve.* Based on lessons gleaned from the experiences of those who came before, health-care ethics provide guidance to members of a healing discipline in:

1. How to create and maintain a vital interpersonal context for providing healing services, and

2. How best to navigate through the various types of challenges that may arise when providing those services.

Along with developing strong professional competence and taking robust care of one's own health and well-being, embracing sound ethical practices is the third pillar for being able to provide outstanding health-care services.

Representing yourself as a practitioner of energy medicine or energy psychology, or any of the more specialized designations within energy healing (a few of the many forms include Reiki, Healing Touch, Therapeutic Touch, Touch for Health, Energy Kinesiology, the Emotional Freedom Techniques, Thought Field Therapy, and the Tapas Acupressure Technique), is a public trust. It assumes you have met the training and practice standards of the appropriate professional organizations and boards and that you demonstrate a commitment to strong professional ethics. This book is designed to help you succeed in that commitment. If an ethics problem arises, the burden of proof is on the practitioner to demonstrate that the actions taken were done in good conscience and informed by the field's established ethical principles and practices.

The *Ethics Handbook for Energy Healing Practitioners* provides practical guidelines for the kinds of ethical issues likely to be faced in an energy healing practice. Because of the alternative status of energy healing and the sensitivities involved in working with the body's energy systems, energy practitioners face ethical challenges that not only fall within but also go beyond the boundaries of conventional healing modalities. As energy healing practices enter mainstream health care, new ethical challenges at the interface of conventional and complementary approaches have also been appearing. For instance, providing energy medicine or energy psychology services to a person in a hospital before and after surgery requires coordination with the medical staff, communication about the purpose and expected effects of the interventions used, and an understanding of institutional sensibilities and lines of authority. The professional subspecialties within energy healing are each represented by one or more organizations, and each of these organizations has addressed ethical issues for its membership in one way or another, sometimes with highly sophisticated ethical codes.

The ethics code presented in this book has been informed by many of those guidelines and codes, and it attempts to present an approach to ethics in energy healing that reflects the highest standards, presented in the most practical manner possible. The *Ethics Handbook for Energy Healing Practitioners* is written to serve the various subspecialties within energy healing, so a given case vignette may be more appropriate for one form of practice than another. We should also emphasize that no single book can cover as complex a topic as professional ethics in a way that addresses the learning needs of every practitioner or that adequately addresses every conceivable ethical dilemma. Additional resources are presented in the references section at the end of the book; there are also instances in which consultation with a colleague, attorney, or your professional organization is the best route for obtaining sound ethical guidance.

In 2024, as the time approached for another printing of this book, we examined its contents to determine if it required updating into a second edition. With hundreds of professionals and paraprofessionals having been required to study the book in order to pass the ethics exams in their respective energy psychology and energy medicine certification programs, it was somewhat amazing that criticisms or concrete suggestions hadn't come our way through the organizers of the various certification programs. But they hadn't. This is in part because we had field-tested and refined the scenarios and the related ethical principles in the Eden Energy Medicine Certification program with more than 1,000 students, many of them already health care professionals, in the five years between the onset of that program and the publication of the book. With that background, and after our most recent review of the content, the volume you are reading is, except for this explanation, unchanged from the original.

A significant gap was, however, apparent at another level than the scenarios and principles laid out in this volume. In the 15 years since the original was written, virtual rather than in-person sessions have become a standard practice. The unique ethical issues raised by online treatment, artificial intelligence, virtual reality, and other electronic communication advances did not fit easily into the structure of this book. We considered adding to this book a section on ethical guidelines about this new frontier in health and mental health service delivery. But it soon became evident that an adequate treatment of these topics requires another book. We invited three well-qualified colleagues—Dawson Church, Anitha Vasudevan, and Kelly Yousem—to take on that challenge and have been consulting with them as the project has developed.

Many principles apply to both volumes, with client welfare generally remaining as the highest priority for all ethical decisions in health and mental health care. However, the devil is in the details. While attempting to strictly follow every item in an ethics code might be an admirable expression of a deep commitment toward the highest standards of health-care service, in the complexities of everyday professional activities, some ethical principles may be unclear for a given situation. Or a sound ethical principle may conflict with another ethical principle, with local laws, or with the expectations of the practitioner's employer. Difficult judgment calls may be required to resolve such conflicts, and there are numerous situations where it may not be possible to follow rigorously every ethics standard published in your profession or in this book. Welcome to the complex world of stepping into another's life with an intention to help! It is as worthy a journey as it is challenging.

We invite other professional organizations to adopt or revise the ethics code presented in this book. You may download this code at no cost and modify it for your organization's purposes according to the guidelines described at *www.EnergyMedicineEthics.com*.

CHAPTER 1

Ethical Dilemmas You May Face

We are, at least in part, drawn into the healing professions because it pains us to see people suffer and we believe that we have tools or gifts that can reduce suffering, enhance health, and promote overall well-being. Leading from that pure and powerful motivation in offering our services to the public, we may nonetheless find ourselves faced with situations where our good intentions are not enough to produce the outcomes we desire for our clients. In fact, despite our purity of intention, we may become embroiled in situations in which our clients feel we have done them harm and question our motivations, and our colleagues judge us harshly. Informing ourselves of our profession's ethical guidelines is one of the most potent steps we can take to avoid such hazards and to navigate safely through volatile circumstances if they do arise.

> To truly serve our clients we need not have just good hearts, but educated hearts.
> —*The Educated Heart, p. 1*

Scope of Practice

Unfortunately, good intentions can sometimes innocently trump sound judgment. A woman is referred to you by her physician who believes her ulcerative colitis can be better treated using an energy and dietary approach rather than by routinely starting her on medication. You learn that she is going through a divorce. After an assessment, your work focuses on her large intestine and spleen meridians, and you teach her simple acupoint tapping techniques to help her manage her stress. You also teach her how to energy test for food. Her symptoms rapidly subside. She then brings in her seven-year-old daughter who began wetting her bed after learning of her parents' impending divorce.

You develop tremendous sympathy for mother and daughter. The husband is a successful attorney whose overwhelming schedule leaves little time for his daughter or for any real family life. He is a harsh disciplinarian when he is present, and both mother and daughter are afraid of him. In the divorce proceedings, he is insisting on financial arrangements that would leave mother and daughter nearly destitute, and he is threatening to obtain custody of the daughter if the wife does not acquiesce. He has shown little interest or affection for his daughter, yet he has made it known that he has built a strong case for obtaining sole custody. In desperation, the mother asks you to testify that in your professional opinion, she will be the better parent. You are pleased to have an opportunity to be a voice for justice in this situation and strongly present sound reasoning that the girl will be better served in her mother's custody. Despite the opposing attorney's attempts to cast doubt on your credentials, the woman wins primary custody as well as a fair financial settlement.

So far so good. Six weeks later, however, you are served with a summons. The husband is suing you for damages as well as registering a complaint with your ethics board that you used your influence improperly in the divorce proceedings. You recommended that custody be awarded to the mother without ever having met, interviewed, or assessed the father. Furthermore, you are not a mental health professional nor do you have specialized training in evaluating custody disputes.

Your sense of outrage about the father's behavior and demands eclipsed your understanding of your "scope of practice." You might have been able to make a legitimate link between what you found in the daughter's energy system and her emotional stress about the divorce, possibly even connecting these with her enuresis, but speculation beyond that took you out onto a very shaky limb. Knowing the boundaries of your areas of competence in the eyes of the law could have helped you move into the situation with your eyes open (enlisting, for instance, a colleague with the proper training and credentials) rather than blindly falling into serious ethical and legal difficulties.

Boundary slip-ups usually have an innocent motivation.
—*The Educated Heart, p. 17*

This unfortunate outcome was avoidable. Most ethical blunders can, in fact, be avoided with basic knowledge of ethical guidelines and a determination to apply them. In this case, the larger issue was your "scope of practice," specifically the boundaries of your credentials and your publicly recognized professional competence. Another bedrock ethical principle has to do with "informed consent" and the "full disclosure" that makes informed consent possible. This can be particularly tricky with energy healing, which is often surrounded by an aura of mystery and magic and may attract desperate people in dire straits.

Informed Consent

Blatant omissions or deceptions in one's disclosure statements clearly constitute negligence, but sometimes in energy healing the issues are so subtle they could never lead to an ethics board taking action against the practitioner. Nonetheless, they may still involve lapses in awareness that do harm. For instance, you have been working for two years with a woman who has become one of your favorite clients. You helped her overcome fibromyalgia, and she continues to consult with you every few weeks for "tune-ups." One day she comes in clearly distraught. She has just learned that she has breast cancer and that it has metastasized. You are shocked. You ask her if she had any signs or warnings. She tells you that she was aware of a lump in her left breast that had been slowly increasing in size, but she was confident that if it were dangerous, you would have detected the malignant energies during her regular visits and warned her.

Most clients already give us more authority than is rightfully ours. It's up to us to stay honest and within the bounds of what we know.
—*The Educated Heart, p. 20*

While this is an extreme case where mind-reading on your part might have been the only way to have prevented a disastrous outcome, you are well advised to explore a client's expectations and beliefs about your powers as an energy healer. Although it is appropriate to express hope and optimism, it is also critically important to be clear and realistic about your personal limitations as well as those of your unconventional profession, particularly when the client is hoping for help with a serious illness.

Unrealistic expectations may also be at play if someone with a particular condition is referred to you because you helped someone else with that condition. The person making the referral may have raved about what you did and how quickly the results were obtained, and your new client may understandably expect the same outcome. Although it is not necessary to dissuade someone of realistic hope, some potential hazards are built into the referral.

> Although we can sometimes relieve a condition that wasn't helped by the usual medical regimen of drugs or surgery, that doesn't mean that we can hang out a shingle that reads, "The Doctor Is In."
> — *The Educated Heart, p. 20*

Say the new client is a man who has severe migraines and you have helped one of his coworkers with occasional moderate migraines. Though you may feel fairly confident that bringing the man's energies into a good balance and flow will help with his migraines as well, you are wise to inform him that no two people's energies are alike, no two people with migraines are alike in what they need, the appropriate treatment for him may be very different from what his friend received, and the results may vary. Otherwise, if his response is slower or less favorable than his friend's, the positive aura he has placed around you may quickly darken into disappointment and unwillingness to cooperate further, or he may sink into a sense of personal failure and despair. The possibility of slower progress was foreseeable and could have been addressed by sensitive full disclosure during the first session.

> Informed consent... means that there should be no surprises for our clients.
> —*The Educated Heart, p. 15*

Overselling your abilities is another hazardous temptation. We all want to put on our best face in our community and in our advertising. Plus, for some clients, there is already a glow of magic associated with those who can work with invisible energies. If these combine to attract clients with life-threatening conditions such as cancer, heart disease, ALS (Lou Gehrig's disease), bipolar disorders, or progressive illnesses such as Parkinson's or multiple sclerosis, you are ethically required to lead the person in realistically distinguishing between their hopes and what you can reliably offer.

Even with less pressing conditions, attributing extraordinary powers to you may undermine a client's self-healing capacities and willingness to participate in self-care. Imagine an older woman who is prone to calling you an "angel" and speaking effusively about your "miracle touch." It may, in fact, be gratifying to bask in her excessively high regard for you. And though you do not need to minimize the skills you have to offer or your importance in her life—your caring and proficiency are indeed gifts to her—you may be fostering a dependence that prevents her from developing her own self-reliance and natural self-healing abilities.

Many of the most advanced healers who are regularly associated with impressive outcomes are inwardly modest and careful not to elevate themselves. They know they are working with forces that are far beyond any one personality or approach and do not take outcomes too personally. You and your clients are best served when you keep your emphasis on their natural self-healing capacities, which you are evoking—placebo effect notwithstanding. This is particularly true with clients who try to attribute magical abilities to you. The more they do this, the more they disempower themselves and the higher your fall in their esteem when they realize you are a mere mortal. Although not a matter of enforceable ethics, challenging extravagant expectations keeps your clients involved in their healing in ways that only make your work with them more potent.

> We don't need to embellish our skills or knowledge. If we do
> what we're trained to do competently and with compassion,
> it's more than enough.
> —*The Educated Heart, p. 19*

Sometimes clients want you to work under conditions that may actually be hazardous to their health. For instance, bipolar disorder (manic-depressive illness) affects more than six million Americans. It is a life-threatening condition that often results in self-destructive behaviors and sometimes in suicide. While existing medications allow many patients to live relatively normal lives, others are not helped or suffer such serious side effects that they elect not to use the available medications. This may lead to desperate situations for the patient and the patient's family and friends. There is a reasonable chance that over the course of an energy healing career, you will be consulted by at least one person with bipolar disorder who wants help in coping without medication. Two serious ethical questions inevitably accompany such a request. First, what can you reliably say about the likely impact of your services on the condition? Second, are you unwittingly conspiring with a person who hates the side effects of the medication to discontinue or not utilize a potentially life-saving though unpleasant treatment? Here your desire to offer hope and help must be carefully weighed against the real dangers in the situation, all discussed in the context of full disclosure and recorded in your case notes.

Conflicts of Interest

Full disclosure involves not only noting the limitations and possible negative effects of the interventions you use, but also potential conflicts of interest. For instance, you host a local television program about energy healing, and it is generating far more referrals than you are able to accept in the large city in which you practice. You are devoting a great deal of time to the program with no direct financial return beyond the referrals, which you do not need, and routing them to other practitioners is, in fact, consuming even more of your time. You decide to make these referrals pay off. You contact the people you consider to be the three best energy healers in the region and propose an arrangement whereby your organization is paid 25 percent of the fee for clients you refer. Two of the practitioners accept. This behind-the-scenes arrangement seems entirely fair to you since you are doing highly effective marketing for these colleagues as well as a service for those who contact you. What are you, in your innocence, neglecting? In providing referrals, you are ethically obligated to keep your clients' well-being as your highest priority. Yet such fee-splitting arrangements give you incentive to refer to the two colleagues who accepted your offer rather than to the third, who did not, regardless of who is the best fit for the client.

> Good boundaries don't occur naturally. They need to be
> studied and practiced in the same way that we learn anatomy,
> physiology, or technique.
> —*The Educated Heart, p. 10*

Conflicts of interest may take many forms, some more blatant than others. For instance, energy testing people for supplements that the practitioner sells for a profit is a widespread practice, used in various alternative healing disciplines. It ignores, however, the potential encroachment of personal gain or even well-intended expectations on the test's objectivity. Or an energy healing practitioner, who after years in the field still does not see or feel subtle energies, purchases a device that is guaranteed to balance the meridians and takes a weekend seminar in how to use it. All his clients are routinely given treatment with this device as part of their sessions. Is it wrong, as better technologies emerge, to use them? Not necessarily. But even if recognized scientific research has established the device as being accurate and effective—a very large "if" at this point—to use it routinely with every client regardless of the person's condition or reasons for seeking energy healing services is itself ethically problematic. It bypasses a comprehensive individual needs assessment—a hallmark of professional practice—and smacks of coercion.

Confidentiality

Confidentiality is another area where uninformed innocence can lead to serious problems. Several "confidentiality traps" may seem obvious after the fact, but consider these common errors: leaving messages on a client's answering machine that may be checked by the client's family members or colleagues, sending e-mails or faxes to devices that may be viewed by others, approaching clients in public to say hello when they may then find themselves having to explain to their acquaintances how they know you, or leaving appointment books open and on your desk in a shared office. Extra vigilance is also required if you take your case notes out of the office. Imagine seeing them in your rearview mirror scattering through a busy street after you placed them on the roof of your car, searched for your keys, and then drove off.

Or consider casually saying to a friend, who had mentioned a person named Bob Oldclient, "Oh, I saw Bob years ago for energy work," and finding out that your friend later said to Bob as a conversation starter, "I think we know someone in common." This could evolve into an unfortunate way of being reminded that confidentiality has no time limit. What if a prospective client says, "My brother came to see you a few months back, right?" She seems to know about it, so you say, "Yes, he did." Later you learn that she and her brother are embroiled in a legal battle and the real purpose of her consultation with you was to verify that he had been spending some of their mutual inheritance on weekly energy sessions with you. Okay, a bit more Machiavellian than what healers usually encounter, but in any case, it is your job to protect your client's private health-care information, including the basic fact of having utilized your services.

> Clients who are friends with other clients may sometimes
> test you to see if you will talk about their friend to them (and,
> therefore, talk to the friend about them).
> —*The Educated Heart, p. 76*

Confidentiality issues may pose eye-crossing ethical challenges even to practitioners who are sophisticated and experienced. Though it might seem straightforward simply to abide by the policy that everything about a client's work with you is strictly protected, situations may arise where it is not so simple. Your informed consent statement can spell out the situations that may be reasonably predicted, but a turn of events may still take you by surprise.

An elderly man has been distraught following the death of his wife of fifty years. In the initial session, he asks about confidentiality and you assure him that his privacy will be protected. He goes on to tell you that his seventy-three-year-old wife had advanced Alzheimer's and he could not stand to see her continued deterioration. He gave her an overdose of sleeping pills and then staged a drowning in the bathtub that was ruled by the authorities to be an accidental death.[1] While this might seem like exactly the kind of case for which confidentiality protection was designed, you may be legally obligated to report the man. In states where child protective laws have been extended to seniors or the handicapped, it is mandatory to report individuals who have intentionally caused the death of a person for

---

1 This case is taken from Koocher & Keith-Spiegel, 2008.

whom they were caring. You may still choose not to report what in the eyes of the law is murder, because you feel this is the higher ethical option. But by not having been explicit about the limits of confidentiality when asked directly, you have placed yourself in a moral dilemma if you decide you do have to report his actions to the authorities. And in any case, you have set up a situation in which he provided you with information he believed was confidential but that the law requires you to report.

> Confidentiality is at the core of professional relationships. It begins with the first phone call.
> —*The Educated Heart, p. 14*

The duty to intervene if your client is placing another person's safety in jeopardy is fraught with confidentiality dilemmas. Some clinicians believe that laws requiring a therapist to step in undermine the entire therapeutic relationship by placing limits on its bedrock confidential nature. They even argue that the intended victim is safer if the person can continue treatment than if a warning is provided and the therapeutic bond broken. The duty to warn is established in the laws of most states, however, and in certain very thorny circumstances, it can provide you with protection even if your client feels violated because you warned a potential victim.

For instance, suppose your client contracted HIV from a woman he loved very much and who died from AIDS a year earlier, two years into their relationship. He is going through a complex grief reaction mixed with anger and confusion. Although your work with him is focused on boosting his immune system, you learn that he has been acting out his anger by having unprotected sex with every woman he can bed. You do everything you can think of to get him to cease and desist, but your pleas do not seem to be landing well. After one of your sessions with him, you jot down your case notes as usual. A couple of minutes later when you step into your waiting room to call in your next client, you see that he is still there and your next client is giving him her phone number along with nonverbal cues of romantic interest. Are you required to warn her using information that was provided to you in confidence? Ultimately, in most states, yes, now that you can identify a potential victim. An entire literature and set of case laws has emerged around this issue (search for "duty to warn" and "HIV"). A first step could be to ask your endangering client to come in for a no-charge session at the first opportunity, or in a phone call, state your dilemma, explain the ethical and legal reasons you must intervene, and seek his permission. If you do not receive it, a quick consultation with a colleague or attorney to be sure you are thinking clearly about your duties and options might be a next step. There will be repercussions no matter what action you take or don't take, and a careful and informed assessment is the best you can do when conflicting ethical principles (duty to warn vs. protecting confidential information) are at play. Ethical behavior is sometimes a compromise within impossible choices.

> The best course of action is not always clear.
> —*The Educated Heart, p. 4*

Other confidentiality dilemmas emerge when more than one member of a family is seeking services. Failure to spell out the lines of communication clearly and in advance can lead to situations in which there is no option that protects everyone's interests, such as if a seventeen-year-old teen confides to you that he has been setting fires and wants your help to control the impulse. Are you obligated to inform his parents, possibly ending the chances of being able to help him by shattering the trust he has placed in you? Your quandaries may be further exacerbated if you have reason to believe that he is considering setting another fire that could jeopardize human life and are required to report this suspected intention to the authorities. Although diligent recording in your case notes of the circumstances, reasoning, dates, and parties involved will not solve the angst if you are faced with such dilemmas, it helps protect you if you reveal confidential information to another party, even if you are required to do so by law.

Legal proceedings may also complicate your choices around confidentiality. Your thirty-two-year-old client was in an industrial accident and is suffering from nightmares and debilitating anxiety as well as the aftermath of physical injuries. In taking her history, you learn that she was treated for anxiety while in college. She is suing her employer for emotional damages and her attorney wants you to testify that her anxiety is debilitating. Can you provide this opinion without revealing, if asked by the opposing attorney, as you likely will be, that there was a preexisting condition (which might undermine her claim)? You need to know the bounds of confidentiality before you take the stand. For instance, once the woman signs a release of confidentiality privileges, allowing you to testify, all the information you have is open. A release of this nature cannot selectively allow certain types of information to be revealed while retaining confidentiality on others.

Clients Who Are Self-Destructive

In addition to the duty to protect others from physical harm, challenges regarding confidentiality emerge if you become aware a client is having suicidal thoughts. Perhaps a woman you have been working with reveals that she has been imagining how much easier it would be to no longer exist and sometimes feels tempted to overdose on prescription pills. The laws of most states require you to take action if you assess that the person is in clear and imminent danger. If you have reason to believe that *thoughts* about suicide have crossed the line into probable *intention,* you are required as the member of the health-care community who has this information to take specific steps that may include the disclosure of information that is otherwise protected.

> Keeping good boundaries is a little like steering a car – it takes constant correction.
> — *The Educated Heart, p. 15*

These steps may include arranging supervision by family or friends and shepherding the person into treatment by an appropriate mental health professional or at least overseeing arrangements for an evaluation in the emergency room of a local hospital or other community resource. You may not have time to do a lot of research when such a case arises, so it is a good idea to prepare yourself in advance for this type of emergency, including maintaining an up-to-date referral network. In cases of immediate danger, a call to 911 may be appropriate.

The line between suicidal thoughts and clear and imminent danger may not be clear-cut. You may be unsure whether a client is truly at risk. Suicidal ideation is a common symptom of depression and trauma and does not necessarily imply *intent* to harm oneself. First of all, even though you are not qualified to assess suicidality if you are not a licensed mental health professional with such training, you can inform yourself about what is known. Considerable research and literature is readily available on the factors that lead to suicide and on assessing serious suicide attempts. For instance, the more a person has thought through a plan and has access to the means to implement it, the greater the risk. A suicide prevention hotline may be able to provide you with references, as can numerous websites. Ultimately, the most responsible step is to enlist the support of a mental health professional through consultation and/or referral, but you may need to make some decisions before completing the session in which suicidal thoughts are revealed to you.

> Practitioners who try to act like counselors are often clumsy— doing things that a good psychotherapist would not do, such as giving advice, confronting clients bluntly, or making hasty interpretations.
> —*The Educated Heart, p. 22*

You can begin by acknowledging the seriousness of what you have heard and informing your client that you want to be sure that his or her feelings and needs are being adequately addressed by those professionals best equipped to do so. You might make a verbal or written contract outlining the immediate concrete steps that will be taken to ensure the person's safety, including a mechanism that keeps you updated about whether the steps are indeed being taken. If your client provides reassurance that he or she is safe from self-harm, and you are somewhat assured, you might still introduce into the discussion that suicidal thoughts point to the need for mental health care. In making the case that your work cannot substitute for a thorough assessment and possible treatment by a mental health professional, be sensitive to the possibility that the client might feel abandoned by you. Emphasize that you will continue to provide your services along with your recommendation of other services. As always, it is important to document in your notes what steps you have taken to act in your client's best interest.

> Honor the dictum, "First do no harm."
> —*The Educated Heart, p. 20*

The need to involve other professionals may also emerge if you see your client's health jeopardized by conditions such as an eating disorder, an untreated infection, or self-cutting. As a general rule, any condition that is potentially life-threatening or is likely to respond better to allopathic medicine than to your services alone will require you to involve other professionals. Though your client has the right to self-determination, you also have an obligation to state when you feel your services are not the best or the only services available to address the problems the client presents. A team approach with multiple providers may be the most efficient and even the most cost-effective way of resolving the client's presenting problem.

Clients Who Are Being Abused

If you notice signs of physical abuse concealed in what you are being told, or appearing on your client's body, your next steps may be particularly delicate. Excessive bruising may be a medical problem, but it may also be suggestive of abuse. A first step would be to state compassionately your concerns, listen to what your client shares in response, and begin discussing what steps need to be taken to build safety. If you are working with a child or a dependent elder, state law may dictate your choices. You may be required to report the signs of abuse to the local Department of Social Services. In many states, you are required to make a report on the basis of suspicion alone. This can put you in a highly uncomfortable position. Your client may beg you not to file a report. You may not be confident that a protective service investigation is going to help the situation. You may feel that breaking the confidence and essentially accusing a caregiver based on insufficient information will cause more harm than potential benefit. If you believe your duty to your client's welfare conflicts with state law, the burden of proof will fall on you to establish this connection. In most cases, the best course is to explain to your client that you are required by law to make the report, empathize with your client's feelings about it, and help the person anticipate and plan for possible consequences.

> Practitioners are mistaken if they think they really are that perfect when clients adore them or that awful when clients are mad at them.
> —*The Educated Heart, p. 57*

In working with adults who are being abused, but the law does not require you to report it, you still have an ethical obligation to your client's safety and well-being. People who are caught in abusive situations do not see an easy way out, and there may not be one. Some victims have been made to believe that they are responsible for the abuse or that if they are "better" somehow, the abuse will stop, or that the abuse is the price they must pay to be with someone they desperately love. Confronting such beliefs may be required if the person is to change the situation, and while referral to a mental health professional is highly appropriate, the abused person may not be interested. You can still provide education about domestic violence, that it cuts across all racial, religious, and socioeconomic boundaries (including high-functioning people of means), and that everyone is entitled to support in protecting their basic human rights. It may take a long time for your client to gather the strength to leave an abusive relationship, as the barriers are real and potentially life-threatening. If the person does come to that decision, you can provide information about available services. Most communities have a safe house or an advocacy center. There is also a national hotline (1-800-799-SAFE). You might also want to educate your client about the "cycle of abuse," in which abusers go through "honeymoon" periods that may make it difficult for the abused to recognize that the relationship is still dangerous.

To summarize the previous discussion, when physical harm to your client or to others at the hands of your client is at issue, you may be required to take steps that are outside the bounds of the normal healing relationship.

Working with People You Do Not Like

You may at times find yourself harboring strong negative feelings about a client, making it difficult to be in the heart-centered space that is conducive to healing work. For example, you may notice that you always dread going to work on Wednesday mornings because you'll be seeing a regularly scheduled client who comes in complaining of the same physical or emotional troubles again and again—troubles you find to be of his own making. You are not feeling your characteristic empathy toward this person. Should you try to push such feelings aside out of a sense of guilt, obligation, or professionalism?

> The intimacy of the work can stir up deep emotional associations.
>
> —*The Educated Heart, p. 1*

Your feelings can actually serve as a form of radar about your client, about yourself, or about your relationship. Taking time to reflect on their meaning can reveal how best to proceed. It is not necessary that you like a person to be helpful in a professional relationship, and when you raise your consciousness about the nature of your dislike, you can often reframe your part of the relationship in ways that reengage your interest, renew your sense of what you need to be doing in the treatment, and even revive your empathy. If self-reflection does not bring clarity, consulting with a colleague, supervisor, or therapist may shed light on unconscious material. We all have blind spots.

Current stresses or other circumstances in your life may be coloring your ability to see the client objectively. Or perhaps the client is triggering feelings in you that belong to unresolved experiences from your past or that push beyond the edges of your own development and comfort zone. Your client may remind you of a parent, ex-spouse, or someone who has bullied you. Your client's issue might be one that is very sensitive for you— such as abuse if you have been abused, or cancer if you have lost a loved one to cancer. There are countless ways our clients can trigger us. If your reaction traces to unresolved issues from your past, recognizing this provides an occasion for working through that issue. Life may be presenting you with another "damned opportunity" for growth.

> If our own boundaries have been violated as children—sexually, emotionally, or physically—then what comes "naturally" to us may be off-kilter.
> —*The Educated Heart, p.6*

It is usually not appropriate, however, to use the relationship with your client directly as the way to confront your own unresolved feelings, but rather recognize that the issue deserves time and focus outside the sessions, with the help of a colleague, supervisor, or therapist if necessary. If you cannot, or choose not to tackle this issue at this point in your life and it is interfering with your giving full measure to the healing process, a referral should be considered.

> Clients need to have a special environment that is focused solely on their well-being.
> —*The Educated Heart, p. 26*

Your strong reaction may, of course, be an appropriate response to the client's manipulation, failure to respect your boundaries, or failure to take responsibility in the healing process. A bit of personal reflection may make it clear where you need to be more forthright in insisting that existing agreements be kept or new ones articulated and entered. Few things taint a healer's empathy more than a client who won't improve due to noncooperation, and getting a new handle on how to confront that noncooperation can bring new life and engagement into the relationship.

If such efforts fail, you may reach a point at which you discuss termination of the sessions. You are, in fact, ethically obligated to discontinue treatment that does not hold promise in addressing the client's needs. Discussing possible termination of the sessions can, however, also be a powerful wake-up call for the client, bringing the noncompliance or self-sabotage into the spotlight. For instance, a client with multiple sclerosis feels much better after every session. You are able to establish a balance between the spleen and triple warmer meridians and to activate the radiant circuits. But try as you might, the person will not follow up with daily maintenance that keeps the spleen meridian strong, and the progress is lost by the next session. So you once more do the repair work, the client feels better, goes home, does nothing, and all ground gained is again lost. As your exasperation grows, you have some choices. You can let it seethe; you can let it fuel ever more creative strategies for trying to get your client to cooperate; or you might eventually draw a line that respectfully and empathically but firmly makes continued treatment contingent on compliance at home. Other ways of undermining treatment, such as frequent missed appointments or "dietary sabotage" of the healing process may call for similarly firm measures.

> We should not work with abusive or disrespectful clients...
> we can decline to work with any client when we do not feel it
> is in our best interests [or theirs] to do so.
> —*The Educated Heart*, p. 15

Sometimes the issue is something about the person that you cannot overlook. You may tell a client who regularly shows up under the influence of alcohol that you will no longer schedule appointments because it is self-defeating for both of you. Or imagine a client who regularly makes racial slurs and derogatory remarks about certain ethnic groups. You believe the person has the cognitive abilities to see the effect this has on others and the ability to monitor this behavior. Despite multiple efforts to address the issue, the remarks appear to be escalating. Do you have a right to terminate an otherwise productive healing relationship on this basis alone?

Your first obligation is to the client's welfare, but if you are feeling verbally abused or physically threatened or coerced, you have every right to terminate the relationship. Discussing other treatment choices and providing referrals is appropriate, though if you are feeling physically threatened, reestablishing a situation that feels safe to you is the first order of business. In the case of the racial slurs, if the continued remarks are rendering you unable to proceed with the rapport needed for you to be fully effective, and you decide to terminate the relationship, the reasons you give may vary with the circumstances. It may not be your place to pass personal judgment on a client's prejudices, but it is certainly your place to speak of your discomfort and how that discomfort was the deciding factor in your decision. In some situations, you may decide it is best not to state your reasons, explaining only that it is a personal decision. Such choices may require a period of reflection and consultation.

> We may think that professional boundaries are just common
> sense, but it's not that simple.
> —*The Educated Heart, p. 6*

If, for any reason, you decide to end a healing relationship that the client would like to continue, the best practice, if at all possible, is to have at least a session or two for review, closure, and discussion of next steps and possible referrals. A sudden unilateral discontinuation of services can leave the client feeling abandoned, unresolved, confused, and less able to trust future health-care providers. It is appropriate only in situations in which you feel physically or emotionally unsafe, are not in good enough health to continue to work effectively, or have had other extenuating life circumstances intervene.

Professional Boundaries

Maintaining the professional boundaries called for in healing work may seem alien or even counterintuitive to people who are accustomed to jobs for which there are no explicit rules about confidentiality, dual relationships, or creating emotional safety. It may feel rude to let a client know that while you value the friendliness of your interactions, you do not answer the kind of personal question that the client just asked in total innocence and trust. It may feel burdensome to have to remain mindful and vigilant about whether a particular self-disclosure will enhance or detract from your work. It may feel ungracious to decline services to someone in your social circle because of the issues around dual relationships or to decline an invitation to a client's retirement party. It may feel restrictive to restrain yourself from chatting with your friends about the details of what you did during your workday. Even if you do not use names, you never know when details you mention might lead someone to recognize the identity of a client.

> Misconception #1: "I want to be natural with clients; boundaries create barriers."
> —*The Educated Heart, p. 5*

Common boundary errors include meeting clients outside your office, engaging in casual phone calls, making yourself available at odd hours, accepting extravagant gifts, or assuming that sharing a great deal about your own issues is an appropriate way of building intimacy. Clients will often become confused and disillusioned if they come to view you as a friend. That perception is not only headed toward bad feelings on the client's part, it also undermines the professional relationship. Clear boundaries allow for predictability and consistency in the healing relationship. They create the safety and trust that support the healing work. Excessive sharing about your own life may detract from the focus on your client, and it may reflect an excessive reliance on your clients for your own needs for connection and care. Having a strong social support network and enjoyable activities outside your professional life will go a long way in supporting appropriate boundaries at work.

Some practitioners unwittingly cross ethical boundaries by asking clients to distribute business cards on their behalf, to help them locate students for classes, or to provide testimonials while still in treatment. The purpose of the relationship is your client's healing. Your fee is the clean, clear medium of exchange. When you add your personal agendas into the mix, they can and often do dilute or confuse the healing work. In addition, the power differential in the relationship can make such requests unintentionally coercive.

> A boundary is like a professional circle around the profes-
> sional relationship that separates what is appropriate from
> what is not.
> —*The Educated Heart, p. 2*

The built-in power imbalance in the professional relationship also means that many clients will not feel comfortable telling you if something is not working for them or if their needs are not being met. Imagine a client who wants to go to the bathroom but is too timid to interrupt the session. Although a boundary around your personal disclosures is important, as discussed, building bridges that allow regular feedback not only prevents absurd situations such as the missed bathroom break, but also provides you with vital information for the healing process.

A few cues from you can help build such bridges. You might say, "It is very helpful when I hear what is going on with clients, so please let me know if anything is uncomfortable for you or if there is anything I can do to make your experience more positive." You can also check with clients at the end of a session by asking what they liked about the session and if anything could have been changed to make it a better experience. You might also signal that you are at ease receiving feedback with statements such as, "You know, some people have told me that they don't like it if I have been completely silent during this procedure; others don't like it if I talk." Regularly reviewing how your client is experiencing the work allows for corrections, better treatment, and happier clients. It is well known that ethical complaints and malpractice suits are less likely to be lodged against doctors who take the time listen to their patients' concerns, acknowledge errors, and take responsibility for their behaviors.

> Good boundaries don't create walls between client and prac-
> titioner; rather, they create a safe space within which we can
> touch clients' hearts and ease their spirits.
> —*The Educated Heart, p. 10*

Paradoxically, in order to honor your primary ethical responsibility—serving the best interests of your clients—you need to prioritize your own self-care. For example, if you keep an appointment with an insistent client at a time when you may be coming down with the flu, you are making it more likely that you will wind up with the flu while providing services that are compromised by your own physical challenge, not to mention putting your client in harm's way. Indications that you need to attend better to your own self-care are feeling regularly exhausted, skipping meals, overlooking your need for time with family and friends, or ignoring basic self-care routines such as exercising and doing your own energy work. Self-care boundary issues that may be involved include over-scheduling yourself, under-charging for your services, working longer with clients than the originally agreed-upon time, or thinking about your clients excessively outside of work hours. Knowing and attending to the signs of burnout or vicarious trauma—occupational hazards for all helping professionals—is another important aspect of keeping yourself healthy.

If your availability to your clients should change for any reason (vacation, new responsibilities, schedule shifts), provide advance notification, address any concerns the client may have, and take measures for the client's continued care, whether a self-care plan or seeking another professional in your absence. Although it is not in your client's interest to foster unnecessary dependence, you have been entrusted to provide consistent care. If you are not able to offer regular appointments, your client should be informed of this before commencing services. Life provides all sorts of challenges and disruptions, but your ethical responsibility is to keep your commitments to the best of your ability. Providing reliable care to your clients means keeping appointments, showing up on time, providing notification far in advance should there be changes, being accessible if additional appointments are needed, preventing disruption during your sessions, and making referrals for coverage while you are away.

> Sessions start and end on time... Nothing interrupts a session.
> —*The Educated Heart, p. 33*

Some boundary problems can be avoided by adhering to well-conceived policies. Suppose you have a client who complains to you that she has heard that someone at her church is getting a lower rate than she is. She is further frustrated by the fact that she just met someone in the waiting room who says she is new to your practice, but just last week you told her she could not refer a coworker to you because you currently have no openings. If you have established clear policies around the issues of serving your clients fairly and consistently, you will be able to respond simply and without defensiveness. You might say, "I cannot comment on other clients' fee arrangements in order to protect their confidentiality, but I am happy to review with you the policy sheet you were provided that covers billing and scheduling. It mentions that I have a limited number of sliding scale slots based on financial need. Also, I keep some slots open for clients who may need to be seen on a more urgent basis because of upcoming medical procedures." Also, you need to think through how you will consistently handle bounced checks, clients whose financial situation changes, and returning clients who may expect to circumvent the waiting list. Having a policy for yourself around these common situations will keep you from having to make spot decisions that may be hard to defend later.

> Three common ways we venture outside the safe boundaries of the professional relationship: bringing in our social and personal needs, going outside our scope of practice and expertise, and mixing our practices with other businesses.
> —*The Educated Heart, p. 17*

Another set of boundary issues involves dual relationships. In small communities in particular, dual relationships may be unavoidable. Your desktop crashes and your client is the only person in town who fixes computers. Can you ask your client to do a home-based repair? The "Ethics Code for Energy Healing Practitioners" attempts to provide guidelines on such decisions, but the client's welfare and the integrity of the healing services you provide are always the *first* considerations. Special challenges around dual relationships may arise if you offer energy healing sessions and also teach energy healing classes in the same community. Clients may come to your classes. Students may wish to become your clients. But the relationship is very different in each of the two situations. You may now be in the position of having to evaluate and pass or not pass a student who is also your client. Or you may find yourself treating your client differently from the other students because you are aware of the person's vulnerabilities, yet you are unable to deal with the discrepancy up front because it involves confidential matters. Or your client feels jealous in having to share you after having enjoyed the sanctity of a private relationship, is embarrassed and secretive about these feelings, and closes down in your individual sessions. Candid discussion is called for before moving from the role of student to client or client to student, and extra attention to the possible hazards is required if both roles are to be engaged simultaneously.

> In dual relationships, the boundaries are already blurred.
> —*The Educated Heart, p.106*

Other boundary issues may involve personal, cultural, and religious differences. Offering a hug at the end of a session may feel to you like a natural and innocent gesture but feel like a boundary violation to some clients. Frank and open discussion about touch is always appropriate in healing work. Cultural or religious issues might involve how healing is understood, the willingness to acknowledge personal problems, the powers attributed to the healer, beliefs about "past lives" and their possible role in current health problems, the influence of forces from the "other side" in the healing process, or the appropriateness of certain techniques. You may want to ask your clients if there are things they want you to understand about their beliefs, background, or life experiences that may have an impact on your work.

The Reliability of Nonconventional Sources of Information

Energy healing practitioners, more than other health-care providers, may rely on nonconventional sources of information. Remote viewing, distant diagnosis, psychic inquiry, past-life regressions, and "reading" subtle energies are not uncommon. Moreover, clients may attribute special importance or reliability to such information, imbuing the practitioner with a level of authority or knowledge that is, in fact, unrealistic. In addition, clients receiving energy work often enter into altered states of consciousness that make them highly suggestible to the tone and content of what you say.

> When we buy into the illusion that we are somehow better
> than the client, we lose our curiosity about the client—and
> we lose our effectiveness.
> —*The Educated Heart, p. 55*

For instance, a client in her first session with you reports a variety of symptoms that she believes are indicative of childhood sexual abuse, though she has no specific memories of having been abused. She asks you to help her ascertain whether she was abused, and by whom. Sensing her distress, you suggest "seeing what comes up" when working on her chakras. Lying on your table as you circle your hand about six inches above her first chakra, she has disturbing images of her uncle while feeling pain in her genital area. You know that, by some estimates, one woman in four was sexually abused during childhood and you have had other clients with similar symptoms whose recall of abuse did not surface until they were adults. You feel it important to validate her experience since members of her family have been denying that she could have been abused. You have an intuitive sense while doing the chakra work that there was, in fact, an abuse history, and you see in your mind's eye an image of a man with red hair. You tell her you believe she was abused and you wonder whether a man with red hair might have been involved. This clinches it. Her uncle has red hair, plus she holds you in such high regard that she takes this as evidence enough to confront her uncle.

You do not hear from her again. Years later, she comes back to you to let you know what a disaster it was for her and her family that she pressed the belief that her uncle had abused her. Only recently did she enter psychotherapy, and during this work had a memory return of her uncle ragefully sending away some neighborhood boys who were molesting her in a toolshed. In her work with you, she had linked the experience of the abuse with the fragmented memory of her uncle's face. She took your validation of this scenario to be an indictment against him and it has been wreaking havoc within her family ever since. Your client's misguided interpretation of the meaning of your work with her might have been avoided or tempered had you been adamant about the limitations of such information.

No psychic, no healer, no doctor, is 100 percent correct in assessments or recommendations, and the further the source information is from actual physical observation, the more suspect. Does this mean that intuitive or psychic information is inadmissible in energy healing? Not at all, but it must be understood and interpreted in context. Such information needs to be presented with strong disclaimers regarding accuracy. Asking the client for feedback with questions such as "Does that resonate with you?" or "Does that feel on the right track?" sends the useful message that you know your clients are the ultimate experts on their own health and experiences. A stance of humble curiosity and openness is appropriate when working with the powerful mysteries of energy and the human body.

* * *

This brief sampling of the kinds of ethical dilemmas you may face during an energy healing practice is designed to encourage you to become informed about the guidelines and practices that have been formulated by dedicated healers who have "walked the walk" before you. The "Ethics Code for Energy Healing Practitioners" presented in this book is reasonably comprehensive, attempting to crystallize the wisdom of generations of healers, with a special focus on energy healing. Rather than confront you with all 118 of the code's specific points at once, this book presents them in a graduated way that allows you to move experientially into them. We begin with thirty-one points that cover many of the most important ethical principles for energy healers to understand.

Chapter 2

Highlights from the "Ethics Code for Energy Healing Practitioners"[2]

The Eden Energy Medicine Certification Program begins by having students sign the following two-page excerpted highlights from the fourteen-page "Ethics Code for Energy Healing Practitioners" (see chapter 4) that they will be required to aspire toward as graduates of the program. Asking new students to study the entire ethics code without adequate experience and context could be overwhelming, while the excerpted highlights orient them nicely to ethical issues. Similarly, we present the highlights here, early in the book, and will introduce additional principles on a case-by-case basis.

ENERGY HEALING PRACTITIONERS...

1. … hold as the highest priority for their professional activities the health and welfare of their clients, students, and others with whom they become professionally involved. All other statements in this document are elaborations upon this principle.

2. … are fully committed to personal integrity, authenticity, and their own ongoing healing and wholesome development in body, mind, and spirit.

---

2 These ethical principles are summarized/excerpted from the "Ethics Code for Energy Healing Practitioners" presented later in this book. For the most current version of this evolving document, visit *www.EnergyMedicineEthics.com*.

3. … strive for professional excellence through ongoing assessment of personal strengths, limitations, and effectiveness.

4. … conduct business and professional activities with integrity, in a professional, honest, and fair manner.

5. … abide by applicable local, state, and national laws governing their health-care services.

6. … perform only those services for which they are qualified, representing their education, certifications, professional affiliations, and other qualifications accurately.

7. … keep themselves current in their field and continually seek to expand their effectiveness as practitioners.

8. … do not diagnose, prescribe, or treat medical disorders unless simultaneously credentialed to do so, making referrals to other health-care professionals when and as appropriate.

9. … respect the inherent worth, dignity, and uniqueness of all people, and the rights of individuals to privacy, confidentiality, and self-determination.

10. … treat clients, students, and colleagues with respect and courtesy, communicating clearly and sensitively regarding issues that affect the services they provide.

11. … respect the professional status of other health-care practitioners.

12. … resist gossip, but rather speak directly with other energy healing practitioners when concerns about their actions arise, making every effort to resolve differences or ethical issues in a frank, respectful, and wholesome manner.

13. … inform prospective clients of the nature and logistics of their potential services clearly and accurately prior to the commencement of those services, appropriately documenting having done so.

14. … discuss with their clients in advance the limitations or potential problems associated with specific procedures before using them.

15. … uphold the confidentiality of those they serve, informing clients in advance of exceptions, such as legal proceedings that require disclosure and the obligation to disclose information that might prevent clear and imminent danger to the client or to others.

16. … build a collaborative relationship with those they serve.

17. … stay alert to factors that might impact the healing relationship, such as a client's becoming overly dependent or being unable to pay for continued services, and generate, with the client, appropriate strategies for addressing such considerations.

18. … avoid dual relationships that might negatively impact the effectiveness of their services.

19. … are aware of the power differences inherent in the professional relationship and do not exploit them.

20. … never enter a sexual relationship with a client.

21. … are sensitive to the potential impact of having a special facility with subtle energies and use this facility only in a manner that is beneficial to the client and with the client's consent.

22. … support their own health and resilience actively so they are at their best as a practitioner and are modeling what they teach.

23. … keep written records as appropriate to their professional function and setting.

24. … seek to promote accuracy, honesty, truthfulness, and dignity in the practice, teaching, science, and art of energy healing.

25. … clarify professional roles and obligations with clients and colleagues and manage conflicts of interest in a manner that avoids exploitation or harm.

26. … keep their agreements and avoid unrealistic or unclear commitments.

27. … who offer educational programs or presentations ensure that the goals of the program have been properly described and are appropriate for the intended audience, and that the programs are run in a manner that accomplishes their stated goals.

28. … who offer educational programs or presentations create a safe and supportive learning environment, prioritizing the welfare of students who participate in training exercises or who volunteer for demonstrations.

29. … who offer educational programs take steps to ensure that graduates of their programs represent the training received appropriately and

with an understanding of the limitations as well as the potentials of the skills they have developed.

30. ... contribute a portion of their professional time for little or no compensation.

31. ... demonstrate a personal commitment to acting ethically; to encouraging ethical behavior by students, supervisees, employees, and colleagues; and to consulting, as appropriate, with others and with their professional association's ethics code concerning ethical problems.

I will promote an awareness of ethics within the health-care community and attest to my willingness to adhere to the full "Ethics Code for Energy Healing Practitioners" and its updates as posted at www.EnergyMedicineEthics.com.

_____   _____
Signature   Date

CHAPTER 3

The Interactive Case Vignettes

Overview

The full "Ethics Code for Energy Healing Practitioners" (chapter 4) covers general principles designed to guide energy healers toward the best practices and highest aspirations of their profession. Following are fifty case vignettes and discussion of their resolution that provides specific direction for applying these principles in the complexities of an energy healing practice.

When you open your practice to the public, you have little control over who will call or walk through the door. The vast majority of the people you encounter will present situations you are well equipped to handle or to refer without incident. The following case vignettes present situations in which your training, intuition, and past experience can best serve you if also informed by the experiences of others who have been down similar pathways.

To get you thinking about and feeling into ethical dilemmas you might plausibly face in your own practice, we have selected fifty case vignettes that demand solutions that may be difficult to reach or implement. In fact, for many of them, no "perfect" solution exists. Instead, competing ethical principles may be at play, such as when the duty to maintain confidentiality competes with the duty to warn of a client's intention to do harm to another person.

Following the list of the fifty vignettes is a section offering six steps for thinking through an ethical dilemma. Each of the fifty vignettes is then presented again, relevant points from the "Ethics Code for Energy Healing Practitioners" listed, and the ethical dilemma analyzed and discussed. We encourage you to think through the vignette before reading the subsequent discussion. The vignettes can also be used in study groups that discuss a vignette and how to handle it before reading the proposed resolution or review and elaborate upon the proposed resolution.

The purpose of the case vignettes is to prepare, not to scare. In the course of an entire career, you might personally come across only a handful of these kinds of ethical dilemmas. But you don't know in advance which ones you will encounter. So thinking through a broad range of dilemmas both helps to prepare you for whatever you might face and shows you steps you can take that will head off avoidable conflicts. Our intention is that by immersing you and your imagination in these deeply human dilemmas and their resolution, you will gain, in a distilled form, a deeper sense of professional ethics than some health-care providers develop through direct experience in twenty years of practice.

Fifty Case Vignettes Involving Ethical Dilemmas

1. One of your closest friends is diagnosed with cancer, and he is going the conventional route involving surgery/chemo/radiation. If it were you, you would start with a month of aggressive energy healing sessions several times per week supported by daily energy healing self-care techniques. How hard do you attempt to persuade him to try this approach? (See discussion on page 40.)

2. Your friend from the previous dilemma decides to postpone the surgery in order to try an energy medicine approach and gets the oncologist to agree to a one-month delay to see what happens. Your friend insists, however, that you are the one who must do the sessions. Although you have worked with this level of illness in the past, you have never worked with someone close to you who has such a serious diagnosis. You are also concerned that you may not be the best practitioner because your emotional involvement and desire to do a good job might get in the way of doing a good job and might get in the way

of knowing when to suggest that more aggressive procedures may be necessary. What do you do? (See discussion on page 42.)

3. Your closest friend within the energy healing community, a relative newcomer, wants you to be her mentor. How does this impact the friendship? Should you do it at all? (See discussion on page 44.)

4. You are seeing a client who has been having anxiety attacks for the past six months, and you are also seeing her husband for digestive problems. During a breakthrough session with the husband, you learn that he has been having a secret affair. It is immediately obvious to you that his wife's anxiety is based on her picking this up at some level, though you have also been working, with some success, on ways her anxiety seems tied to her childhood history as well as problems with triple warmer and bladder meridians. Can you continue to see her as a client? Him? Could you have taken any steps to prevent this crisis in confidentiality? (See discussion on page 46.)

5. You are teaching a one-evening energy healing class. During the break, a man comes up to you and tells you he has been having energy healing sessions with a practitioner you have not met. He feels the practitioner has made several mistakes in the way he has been treated, which he describes, and asks your opinion. What do you say? (See discussion on page 48.)

6. You refer a client to a chiropractor for some structural work. You have several insights about the relationship of your client's emotions, energies, and structural problems. You have shared some of these observations with him but have not felt he would be able to hear your thoughts about the role of his emotions in his physical problems. Can you share your speculations with the chiropractor? (See discussion on page 49.)

7. You are working with a new client and you sense an energy in the second chakra that feels to you like the energy of cancer. What do you do? (See discussion on page 50.)

8. You are extremely attracted to one of your clients, whom you have had three sessions with and are continuing to see weekly. You find yourself looking forward to this client's sessions and fantasizing about a personal relationship. What actions do you take in response to your feelings? (See discussion on page 52.)

9. Your client is being treated by a physician who is prescribing medication that you believe is both unnecessary and an obstacle rather than an aid to recovery. What do you do? (See discussion on page 56.)

10. A woman who has discovered a lump on her breast does not want to have a biopsy. She comes to you and asks you to use energy testing and intuition to determine if it is malignant. What do you do? (See discussion on page 58.)

11. Your client's physician wants her to stop seeing you because the physician believes that energy healing is quackery and might even do his patient harm. Meanwhile, the patient has not been able to find scientific evidence that energy healing is a legitimate treatment approach and is inclined to follow the physician's advice. But you know your sessions with the client are just starting to have an impact and believe it would be detrimental to terminate them. What do you do? (See discussion on page 60.)

12. You have just completed a powerful regression session and you learn that the client has a Rolfing session scheduled that evening. You are concerned that the Rolfing might prevent an integration of the regression work and might even be harmful. Can you ask a client to reschedule a session with another practitioner? (See discussion on page 62.)

13. You are working your client's neurolymphatic points. Your client is clearly in considerable discomfort. How do you determine if you are applying too much pressure? If you determine the pressure is therapeutic, do you ignore your client's discomfort? (See discussion on page 64.)

14. You are a female working with a male client's neurolymphatic points and have come to the pubic bone. His penis is covering some of the points. What do you do? (See discussion on page 65.)

15. A man who has heard of your ability to sense energies asks you to assess whether he needs a colonoscopy, a procedure that was routinely recommended because he has just turned fifty. You have a very clear perception from sensing his energies, as well as from energy testing, that he does not require a colonoscopy. What do you do? (See discussion on page 66.)

16. A man consults you after his wife is diagnosed with lung cancer. He had been a smoker for the thirty years of their marriage and she had

complained about this for thirty years. He gave up smoking immediately after her diagnosis, and his guilt is enormous. The wife is interested only in a conventional medical approach. He wants to pursue every possible avenue to help her and has heard that energy healing can be done on a remote basis. You ask for her consent, but he begs you to "just do it" because she already has too much on her mind and introducing her to such a strange concept might overwhelm her. Can you do the healings for her without her explicit permission? (See discussion on page 66.)

17. You have been developing your ability in remote viewing and surrogate healing. You have a session with a young man in a few hours and have been thinking about his case. Can you "tune in" to him as you consider how you can best serve him? (See discussion on page 68.)

18. Your client has brought in a medication that has just been prescribed and wants you to energy test it. You find that it tests weak. How do you explain this finding to your client? (See discussion on page 70.)

19. Your client is having terrible PMS. You have several herbal remedies and you energy test them, showing that one in particular tests very strong. Do you recommend that she go to the health food store and purchase it? Do you energy test for a product that you, yourself, sell? (See discussion on page 71.)

20. Your client comes in reporting that she is very unhappy with the treatment she has been receiving from you. She has been doing everything you have recommended and her original condition has not improved after five sessions. The two of you are unable to come to an understanding. The client wants a refund and an apology. You feel you have been following protocol, are puzzled by the lack of response, and do not know the next step. What do you do? (See discussion on page 73.)

21. You receive an e-mail from someone in another region asking you for advice on how to use energy medicine with a specific condition. The person has read Donna Eden's book *Energy Medicine,* watched several DVDs, is trying to self-treat, and found you on a Web listing of energy healing practitioners. What are your responsibilities? Must you respond at all? If so, how soon? (See discussion on page 75.)

22. Your client has a growth that you believe may be malignant. Your client refuses to get a medical diagnosis. You are deeply concerned and feel

the situation is urgent. You plead and cajole. Your client still refuses. You know your client's doctor's name and your client's spouse. What are your responsibilities? (See discussion on page 76.)

23. You wake up with a bad stomachache and a mild temperature. You have five clients scheduled this day, including one who has traveled a considerable distance to see you. What do you do? (See discussion on page 77.)

24. You know that one of the faculty members has been telling a friend who is also a student in an energy healing certification program what is going to be covered on the graduation exam. What do you do with this information? What do you do when you know another energy healing practitioner has committed an ethical violation? (See discussion on page 78.)

25. You intuitively sense that a particular certified practitioner is deeply troubled and that this is compromising the person's work. While you have no direct information that the practitioner is not doing a good job, another member of the community heatedly mentions a concern about this same practitioner. Do you share your intuitive hit? (See discussion on page 79.)

26. At this point (continuing #25), a student in one of your classes asks if you recommend that he schedule a session with the practitioner in question. You have no direct knowledge that the practitioner is not providing good services. How do you respond? (See discussion on page 81.)

27. You are present when several of your energy healing colleagues are discussing their concerns about the treatment choices a specific practitioner has been making. To your knowledge, these concerns, though they seem legitimate to you, have not been shared with the practitioner. Do you immediately turn the person in to the appropriate ethics committee or send an e-mail to the entire energy healing community warning them about this practitioner? Or do good ethics require that you do both? Or neither? Just what do you do? (See discussion on page 82.)

28. You have an intense session with a new client, which includes substantial neurolymphatic work. The next day the client calls you. She feels terrible, is running a 102-degree temperature, believes your session is

responsible for it, and wants you to come right over to her home to give her a free session to treat the aftermath of your original session. What do you do? (See discussion on page 85.)

29. When doing an energy session with a male client, a female practitioner becomes aware her client has a noticeable erection. What would be an appropriate and ethical way to deal with this? (See discussion on page 88.)

30. In a phone interview before a first session with a woman who is seeking help for fibromyalgia, you suspect that she may have a mental disorder or an addiction to illicit drugs. You have no special training, background, or license to treat addictions or serious psychological problems. How should you proceed? (See discussion on page 90.)

31. While at a local restaurant in your small town, you overhear two energy healing practitioners discussing a client. Even though they don't reveal a name, you recognize by the description of the problem the person they are discussing. What are you obligated to do? (See discussion on page 92.)

32. After meeting with a client several times, you are asked to attend a Worker's Compensation hearing regarding a disability the client is claiming. Even though your case notes from a few months earlier did not comment on various issues relevant to the hearing, you feel confident that you can reconstruct your notes, adding pertinent details for the benefit of the hearing. Should you do this? (See discussion on page 94.)

33. After seeing a client for more than a year, you feel satisfied with her progress and feel you have little more to offer. When you talk to the client about ending your work together, she becomes very upset and you learn that she has a strong emotional attachment to you and wants to continue to work with you. What do you do? (See discussion on page 96.)

34. You have a session with a client who has just left an abusive husband and is living in a safe house. Her fears, memories, and physiological reactions quickly surface and become a central part of your work together. You find that you are strongly triggered by feelings from some old personal history around similar issues. How should you proceed? (See discussion on page 99.)

35. You feel good about your client's progress and the work you are doing together. The client expresses feeling great compassion and caring coming from you. A few sessions later, the client admits to feeling a strong romantic attraction toward you. You explain a bit about transference, but later you find that the discussion has sparked your own romantic interest. You are both single and available. Can you become friendlier and continue to work together? Should you refer the client to another practitioner so that you can pursue a personal relationship? Is there any reason you should not explore an opportunity for a meaningful relationship? (See discussion on page 101.)

36. You are deeply involved in working with a woman who has multiple sclerosis and her physician is impressed with the results. The woman's brother has been driving her to the sessions and you have been enjoying brief chats before and after the sessions. The brother invites you to lunch, with clear romantic overtones. You are both unpartnered, and you are interested. Can you pursue this relationship? If your attraction is very strong, but you decide you cannot simultaneously treat the woman and pursue the relationship, can you refer the woman to another practitioner? (See discussion on page 105.)

37. Your client reveals after your third session together that he was a victim of ritual abuse that is still a source of trauma and anxiety for him. In the next session, he has an overwhelming flashback and dissociates. You manage to help stabilize him, but the issues are clearly not resolved. You learn that he has never had therapy for these experiences, but when you recommend therapy, he claims that the cost of both entering psychotherapy and continuing to see you would be prohibitive. You have been helping him with symptoms of hypertension and overall well-being. What do you do? (See discussion on page 107.)

38. You attend a monthly meeting of local holistic health-care providers. You become aware that one of the members has recently added the credential of "MD" to his business card and advertising. When you inquire about the medical degree, he explains that he earned this credential from an East Indian university that offers an online medical degree, the only requirement of which is to write a twenty-five-page paper on the history of miraculous healing. A month later, you have a client who discusses her need for a new MD, says she heard about the

member of your group, and asks you for a referral or an opinion. She wants a medical doctor who has a holistic orientation. What is your responsibility if any to your client, to the practitioner, to the group, and to the community? (See discussion on page 109.)

39. A seventeen-year-old male has contacted you as a result of an article about energy healing mentioning your services, which he saw in a local alternative health newsletter. After making a preliminary appointment, he arrives with his mother. The mother, who will be paying for the session, insists on being present during the session. The young man is clearly giving signs he does not wish that arrangement. What do you do? (See discussion on page 112.)

40. A landscaper calls for an initial appointment. He has been off the job for the past three months due to an injury that is to be a focus of your work together. Once you tell him your fee, he says that he simply does not have the money but he really wants to work with you. He asks if he can do a work exchange of landscaping in repayment for sessions. You have just moved to a new home that needs landscaping. What do you say? Or what if the injured person is a single parent working for low pay at a nursing home, has no savings or health insurance, and can't possibly pay any appreciable fee, but the person can't function adequately without help for the injury? (See discussion on page 114.)

41. A twenty-two-year-old woman who has been responding well in your sessions quite abruptly becomes depressed for no identifiable external cause. Work with homolateral repatterning, neurovasculars, triple warmer, and stomach meridian yields only temporary relief after three intensive sessions focusing on the depression. Are you obligated at this point to refer to a mental health professional for a psychiatric assessment of the depression? (See discussion on page 118.)

42. You are invited to teach in another community. While there, your students complain that an energy healing practitioner who has previously taught in the area did not stay within the announced topic of "energy medicine" and actually taught some "far out" material that a few people liked, but many of the health providers attending felt was unfounded and inappropriate. They ultimately left with a negative impression of energy medicine. You and the other practitioner are part of the same professional association. How do you handle these complaints? (See discussion on page 119.)

43. After a powerful first session, your very ill client describes the session to her minister and calls you to cancel further sessions unless you can assure her that the healing is coming from Jesus and is not the devil working through you. You sense that she is feeling very vulnerable, with her own healing at stake, and caught between two authorities. What do you do? (See discussion on page 122.)

44. You use a product that has given you tremendous health benefits. You feel so strongly about it that you want to make it available to others. Is it ethical for you to sell this product to your clients? If you do not personally sell the product, is it ethical to energy test whether or not your client should use this product? (See discussion on page 124.)

45. An energy healing colleague is in a new relationship and asks for your advice about a dilemma that has arisen. As she begins describing the situation, you realize that her new partner is one of your clients. What should you do? (See discussion on page 126.)

46. An energy healing colleague who is part of your professional association reveals that she has entered into a sexual relationship with a client. She is thrilled with this development. Are you obligated to report her to your ethics committee? (See discussion on page 128.)

47. An energy healing colleague reveals that she has entered into a sexual relationship with a client. She is agonizing about this development and seeking your counsel. Are you obligated to report her to the ethics committee of her professional association? (See discussion on page 130.)

48. In working with a minor child, you suspect that there is some form of abuse currently taking place. How do you handle this with the child? If the child confirms your suspicions, what do you do then? What do you do if the person bringing the child for the appointments is the suspected abuser? (See discussion on page 131.)

49. You attend a lecture in which an energy healing practitioner takes credit for other people's ideas, presenting them as her own. Is this an ethical problem? How should you handle it? (See discussion on page 133.)

50. You have a female client who loves dogs and dog shows. She's a wonderful person who would love to be in a relationship. You have another client who shows his dogs regularly and is also single. You're sure they would be great for each other. What do you do? (See discussion on page 134.)

Six Steps for Thinking Through an Ethical Dilemma

In the complexities of serving in the healing and evolution of fellow human beings, ethical dilemmas cannot be avoided. They are to be expected. Familiarity with the *Ethics Code for Energy Healing Practitioners* orients you toward preventing ethical dilemmas where possible and meeting those that cannot be avoided with clarity, competence, and a spirit that promotes the best interests of all involved. When faced with an ethical dilemma, the following six steps are designed to help you think through the actions you will ultimately take.

1. Recognize that your very human responses in facing this challenge will shape the way you meet it. Mindfully notice your own sensations, emotions, thoughts, judgments, images, memories, or other aspects of your response to the situation. Meet each with your breath and accept that they are at the moment part of your internal landscape. Inquire more deeply as you are moved to do so. Recognize also and accept that there may be no easy or even "right" answer.

2. Comb the *Ethics Code for Energy Healing Practitioners* to identify the basic principles that apply to the situation. While they might not give you the solution, you will know that you are thinking within a sound ethical framework.

3. Gather information. Talk to the other parties involved while staying alert about keeping privileged information confidential. List the critical issues and evaluate the rights, responsibilities, and welfare of the people who will be affected by the actions taken. As the situation unfolds, check in regularly to your shifting internal landscape and allow it to inform you. A good mantra is "Notice breath; soften belly; open heart."

4. Evaluate possible courses of action. If two ethical principles seem contradictory, consider each route independently before finalizing a plan. The overriding considerations are the welfare of your client and all others involved.

5. Obtain consultation as appropriate.

6. Map out the best possible course of action, anticipate possible consequences and steps to minimize harm, decide who needs to be informed, and implement.

The following discussion of the case vignettes presented earlier begins by identifying the ethical principles that are involved. Of the 118 points in the *Ethics Code*, the most relevant for each case are identified and listed. In addition to opening the discussion with well-formulated principles, this also helps familiarize you, in bite-sized quantities, with the points in the Code. The discussion then helps you think through how to apply the principles to come to the best conceivable solutions given each situation.

Discussion of the Case Vignettes

Case Vignette 1

One of your closest friends is diagnosed with cancer, and he is going the conventional route involving surgery/chemo/radiation. If it were you, you would start with a month of aggressive energy healing sessions several times per week supported by daily energy healing self-care techniques. How hard do you attempt to persuade him to try this approach?

Thinking It Through

This is your friend. He is in a situation in which you have special knowledge and expertise. But your orientation is outside the mainstream, and he has elected to put his life into the hands of a more conventional approach. You would like to offer the benefit of your experience. Relevant guidelines include:

1. You take steps to ensure that your personal biases do not negatively impact your services. *(Personal and Interpersonal Boundaries—1)*

2. In deciding whether to provide services to those already receiving health services elsewhere, you consider the health-care issues and the prospective client's welfare carefully. You discuss these issues with the client in order to minimize the risk of confusion and conflict, consult with the other service providers when appropriate, and, in a spirit of respect and cooperation toward all related parties, proceed with sensitivity to the health-care issues involved. *(Informed Consent—3)*

3. You recognize the limitations and subjective nature of nonconventional ways of assessing the flow within a person's energy system. *(The Healing Relationship—11)*

4. You may attempt to encourage but do not attempt to pressure or coerce a client into any action or belief. *(The Healing Relationship—3)*

5. You hold as the highest priority the health and welfare of your client. *(General Principles—1)*

6. You build a collaborative relationship with those you serve and are obligated to respect the other's self-determination. *(General Principles—7)*

7. If conflicts occur regarding your ethical obligations (as in this case, where your belief that your friend's welfare can best be served via energy healing may come into conflict with respecting your friend's self-determination), you attempt to resolve these conflicts in a responsible fashion that avoids or minimizes harm. *(The Healing Relationship—15)*

You have an established, close relationship with this person. But you are also a health-care professional, and a life-threatening situation has arisen in which you are moved to set aside customary boundaries between friendship and your professional role, hoping to bring your expertise into the mix.

You certainly may inquire about your friend's mindset and emotional state regarding the cancer diagnosis and planned treatment. It could, in fact, be very useful to help him to review, evaluate, and analyze what his doctors have told him. You might also help him think through some of the critical questions he may still need to ask: How urgent and aggressive is the cancer? Is the timing of the proposed surgery due to medical urgency, doctor availability, or other factors? Is the proposed treatment the *only* protocol or just the one that is most frequently used? Have other patients of this doctor pursued complementary options? Does the oncology unit where the treatment will occur offer any complementary services?

These questions help him define and envision how he wants to participate in his treatment and healing. Sometimes when a serious diagnosis is announced, the doctor's recommendations are heard as more absolute than even the doctor intended. Posing good questions may show the person that more choices are available than were initially recognized. So far, you are only being a good friend, informed perhaps by your professional experience.

Depending upon how this discussion unfolds, it may be entirely appropriate to ask if he is interested in hearing more about how the work you do might be of benefit to him. If he expresses interest, you could share any first- or second-hand knowledge you have about people who were able to turn around cancer in its early stages using energy healing protocols. Using appropriate disclaimers, you could discuss how you believe this works and fill him in further about energy healing and your experiences with it.

You could also refer him to energy healing materials, such as "Six Pillars of Energy Medicine" (relatively academic, *www.EnergyMedicinePrinciples.com*) or Dr. Christiane Northrup's more personal explanation in her foreword to *Energy Medicine for Women* (free download from *www.EnergyMedicineForWomen.com*), so he could better understand how energy healing works.

If he asks what you would do in the same situation, you are free to tell him, though even here, some caveats are called for. You might say something along the lines of: "Though it is impossible to predict, I believe that I would immediately begin applying energy healing protocols on myself and enlist the aid of other energy healing practitioners to see if we could turn it around before looking to more invasive procedures."

The ethical issue here is at the line between providing information that has been requested or is at least being consensually received versus badgering him or pushing hard to persuade. Although he is not your client, his autonomy is entitled to the same respect as a client's. Particularly if you are advising him to postpone established medical procedures, even if as a friend rather than as a professional, you are taking on an enormous responsibility.

A line should definitely be drawn anywhere that your friend expresses resistance to hearing more or to considering your recommendations. It is yours to try to open a door and provide requested information and ideas. It is not yours to try to push your friend through that door.

CASE VIGNETTE 2

Your friend from the previous dilemma decides to postpone the surgery in order to try an energy medicine approach and gets the oncologist to

agree to a one-month delay to see what happens. Your friend insists, however, that you are the one who must do the sessions. Although you have worked with this level of illness in the past, you have never worked with someone close to you who has such a serious diagnosis. You are also concerned that you may not be the best practitioner because your emotional involvement and desire to do a good job might get in the way of doing a good job and might get in the way of knowing when to suggest that more aggressive procedures may be necessary. What do you do?

Thinking It Through

Your friend has decided to try a round of energy healing but is only willing to work with you. You are concerned that the personal relationship will make you less effective. Additional ethical guidelines include:

1. You do not enter into a dual relationship that might impair your objectivity, competence, or effectiveness in the delivery of healing or educational services. (*Personal and Interpersonal Boundaries—13*)

2. If you enter a dual relationship, you take responsibility to ensure that each party is aware of issues related to shifting between the client-practitioner setting and the social setting of the personal relationship. (*Personal and Interpersonal Boundaries—14*

3. You clarify professional roles and seek to manage conflicts of interest to avoid exploitation or harm. (*Personal and Interpersonal Boundaries—2)*

4. You recognize the pitfalls of being overly attached to the outcomes of the services you provide. Becoming overly invested may have a paradoxical effect. (*The Healing Relationship—6)*

5. You stay sensitive to differences in power between the practitioner and client and do not exploit such differences. (*Personal and Interpersonal Boundaries—10)*

6. You consult with, refer to, or cooperate with others professionals and institutions, with your client's consent, to the extent needed to serve the best interests of the client. (*The Healing Relationship—8)*

First, you would carefully evaluate the alternatives. Is another local practitioner available that you could recommend with confidence? If so, you should at least inform your friend of this option. If he still insists upon seeing you or no one, or if there is no viable referral, you have to weigh the costs and benefits as well as potential strategies for minimizing the disadvantages of a dual relationship. This would be an appropriate time to discuss the situation with a colleague. In particular, examine your own need (as well as the external pressures) to rescue your friend and the complications this can cause. You cannot rescue a person. You can provide the best services of which you are capable, but you cannot control what the outcome of those services will be. The greater your need for a particular outcome, the more your judgment is likely to be clouded as difficult treatment choices emerge.

If you do proceed, you might put temporary boundaries on the friendship for the duration of the time you work together professionally. This might include limiting the relationship to the sessions and might even include charging for your professional time to make it very clear to both of you that the nature and purpose of your relationship has undergone a massive shift.

Ongoing consultation with a colleague would also give you an important sounding board for managing such issues as your need to rescue your friend, the pressure you may be feeling to produce results within the allotted month, finding the line between providing hope and pressuring your friend to "get better," ensuring that your exploration of the factors causing the illness does not devolve into blaming the person for having become ill, and brainstorming decisions such as when it might be necessary to call for more aggressive measures.

CASE VIGNETTE 3

Your closest friend within the energy healing community, a relative newcomer, wants you to be her mentor. How does this impact the friendship? Should you do it at all?

Although taking on a friend as a client is quite different from mentoring a friend, many of the same principles still apply. Pertinent guidelines include:

Thinking It Through

1. You do not enter into a dual relationship that could reasonably be expected to impair your objectivity in the delivery of educational services. *(Personal and Interpersonal Boundaries—13)*

2. If you enter a dual relationship, you take responsibility to ensure that each party is aware of issues related to shifting between the client-practitioner setting and the social setting of the personal relationship. *(Personal and Interpersonal Boundaries—14)*

3. You are sensitive to differences in power between the practitioner and the client and do not exploit such differences. *(Personal and Interpersonal Boundaries—10)*

4. You clarify professional roles and obligations and seek to manage conflicts of interest to avoid exploitation or harm. *(Personal and Interpersonal Boundaries—2)*

5. You recognize that "trying too hard," micromanaging a client, or becoming overly invested may have a paradoxical effect. *(The Healing Relationship—6)*

6. If you find that a potentially harmful dual relationship has arisen, you take "reasonable steps" to resolve it with due regard for the best interests of the affected person and maximal compliance with the "Ethics Code for Energy Healing Practitioners." *(Personal and Interpersonal Boundaries—15)*

You might first look for other possible mentors, and if candidates are available, ask your friend if there is any reason for you to be the mentor that outweighs the potential for complications. If you do proceed, the boundaries here can have more flex than in a formal practitioner-client relationship, but the situation still carries some dilemmas.

The most basic understanding for giving this arrangement the chance to succeed is that your friendship has to take the backseat. When working in this capacity, you are teacher-student first and friends second. Payment arrangements for the mentoring services need to be established. If you still do get together as friends, clear boundaries need to be set about discussing mentoring material at those times. You should also establish an advance agreement that the mentor relationship will be terminated if problems based in the dual relationship arise that the two of you cannot resolve.

CASE VIGNETTE 4

You are seeing a client who has been having anxiety attacks for the past six months, and you are also seeing her husband for digestive problems. During a breakthrough session with the husband, you learn that he has been having a secret affair. It is immediately obvious to you that his wife's anxiety is based on her picking this up at some level, though you have also been working, with some success, on ways her anxiety seems tied to her childhood history as well as problems with triple warmer and bladder meridians. Can you continue to see her as a client? Him? Could you have taken any steps to prevent this crisis in confidentiality?

Thinking It Through

You are caught by surprise and are in a terribly awkward position. Guidelines to consider include:

1. Your client's health and welfare are the highest priority in your professional activities. (*General Principles—1*)

2. Your client is the only person who has the right to determine who has access to information about the energy healing services he or she has received from you. (*Confidentiality—1*)

3. If conflicts occur regarding your ethical obligations, you must attempt to resolve these conflicts in a responsible fashion that avoids or minimizes harm. (*The Healing Relationship—15*)

4. You do not enter into a dual relationship that could reasonably be expected to impair your effectiveness in the delivery of healing services. (*Personal and Interpersonal Boundaries—13*)

5. If you are working with more than one member of the same family, you must establish from the outset the kinds of information that may be shared and with whom, and the kinds of information that may not be shared. (*Confidentiality—2*)

6. You seek to promote accuracy, honesty, and truthfulness in your communications and in the practice, teaching, science, and art of energy healing. (*General Principles—4*)

Even if a clear understanding about the bounds of confidentiality had been achieved, this could be a very difficult situation.

To avoid situations like this, some health practitioners, if treating more than one adult member of the same family, make it clear and explicit with each person involved that any information voluntarily revealed by one family member can be shared with the others. Then each client has a choice and knows in advance that anything they choose to disclose may be shared. Other health practitioners take just the opposite approach, maintaining a seal of confidentiality with each client, even those who are in an intimate relationship or in the same family with another client. Some health practitioners, particularly some psychotherapists, will not treat more than one person in the same family, in part to prevent situations like this one.

The wording of this case suggests that confidentiality for each party was either established or implied. If ever there were an ethical dilemma where there is no "right" answer, this is a strong candidate.

The place where you can start without confusion about what you can say without breaking confidentiality is with the husband. You can explain your ethical dilemma to him. Presuming that his wife's symptoms of anxiety have been shared knowledge among the three of you, you could present your belief that his wife is at some level aware of his affair, that this is contributing to her symptoms, and that the situation puts you into an ethical dilemma as long as you are continuing to work with her on that anxiety. Possible outcomes include that he might choose to tell her about the affair, might end the affair, might separate from her with the intention of getting counseling or of ending the marriage, or he might insist that it is your ethical obligation to maintain confidentiality.

If he opts to insist on confidentiality, or if you have decided not to discuss the situation with him, your choices include:

- You could continue to work with them both and compartmentalize the information. However, should the wife learn that you were told about the affair, she may perceive you as being complicit with the husband in concealing it. This would likely violate her sense of trust and could undermine future work with her.

- You could tell him that though you will not break confidentiality, you will need to tell his wife that for reasons you cannot disclose, you are not able to continue to work with them both and you must refer her to another practitioner. If he still refuses to disclose the affair, you would follow through on this. Your rationale could vaguely include that it is not turning out to be workable to have them both as clients.

- Or you could tell him that the next step is to tell her that you believe the couple dynamics are contributing to her anxiety and that you would like to refer them for couples therapy as a required adjunct to your continued work with her, or as an alternative to your continued work with her.

You would do well to discuss each of these or other options (such as breaking the confidentiality—an option that is hard to imagine choosing) with a colleague and to consider very carefully the possible outcomes of each course of action open to you, based on everything you know about each partner.

Case Vignette 5

You are teaching a one-evening energy healing class. During the break, a man comes up to you and tells you he has been having energy healing sessions with a practitioner you have not met. He feels the practitioner has made several mistakes, which he describes, and asks your opinion. What do you say?

Thinking It Through

Your opinion is being enlisted about a practitioner you have not met by a student who is describing complaints about the practitioner. Relevant guidelines:

1. You hold, as the highest priority, the health and welfare of your clients, students, and others with whom you become professionally involved. *(General Principles—1)*

2. You seek to promote accuracy, honesty, truthfulness, and dignity in the practice, teaching, science, and art of energy healing. *(General Principle—4)*

3. You treat colleagues with dignity, respect, and courtesy; resist gossip; and talk about colleagues in respectful ways. *(Personal and Interpersonal Boundaries—12)*

The ethical guidelines ask you to treat colleagues with respect. Passing judgment on another practitioner's choices without having yourself been involved is a highly questionable move. There are many ways to work toward the same outcome within energy healing. You did not assess this individual and you are not privy to the practitioner's reasoning. So for you to pass judgment, based on this brief conversation, that the practitioner had made "several mistakes" would be highly ill-advised.

You could, however, turn this into a learning opportunity for your student. Articulating some of the previous (e.g., there are many ways to work toward the same outcome) could be quite instructive. You could also encourage the student to talk directly to the practitioner to express his concerns. This could deepen the relationship or uncover irreconcilable differences within it. If your student has attempted or does attempt a frank discussion with the practitioner and remains dissatisfied, seeking another practitioner would be a logical next step.

> **Caveat:** If the "mistakes" presented are of an obvious and gross nature, or violate ethical guidelines, you might be ethically bound to intervene (see *The Resolution of Ethical Issues—1, 2*).

Case Vignette 6

You refer a client to a chiropractor for some structural work. You have several insights about the relationship of your client's emotions, energies, and structural problems. You have shared some of these observations with him but have not felt he would be able to hear your thoughts about the role of his emotions in his physical problems. Can you share your speculations with the chiropractor?

Thinking It Through

You have thoughts about your client's structural problems that are highly speculative. You are not sure how appropriate it is to share these with another professional who is operating within a different paradigm. Relevant guidelines include:

1. You hold, as the highest priority, the health and welfare of your clients, students, and others with whom you become professionally involved. *(General Principles—1)*

2. You treat clients, students, and colleagues with dignity, respect, and courtesy. *(Personal and Interpersonal Boundaries—12)*

3. Your client is the only person who has the right to determine who has access to information about the energy healing services he or she has received from you. *(Confidentiality—1)*

When referring a client to another practitioner, the standard sequence is to provide the client with the practitioner's name and contact information and, except in unusual circumstances, to expect the client to initiate the contact. It is also customary at that point to get a signed release of information that allows you to be in contact with the practitioner about the client. You may then let the practitioner know that you have made the referral along with some basic information about the reason for the referral.

It is also customary to provide the other practitioner with your perceptions about the client, but many practitioners arrange for that discussion only after the initial session so as to allow the practitioner a fresh view of the client. Then concerns, questions, and insights may be shared between the practitioners.

Regarding what would be appropriate for an energy healing practitioner to share with another professional who does not operate from the same framework, your beliefs about the relationship of the client's emotions, energies, and structural problems are appropriate to share. But assuming you do not have laboratory tests or other hard evidence that establishes these relationships, the language you use should acknowledge the speculative nature of your thoughts. It is also your responsibility and your challenge to use language that bridges the alternative paradigm of energy healing with conventional paradigms in order to facilitate respectful communication, understanding, and collaboration among the professionals involved in the client's welfare.

CASE VIGNETTE 7

You are working with a new client and you sense an energy in the second chakra that feels to you like the energy of cancer. What do you do?

Thinking It Through

Energy healing practitioners are not legally permitted to diagnose or treat medical disorders unless specifically licensed to do so. Your training involves assessing and balancing the body's energies and energy systems and educating the client to do so on a self-help basis. If you suspect or have reason to believe your client has a dangerous health condition but does not know about it, guidelines to consider include:

1. You do not diagnose or treat illness unless you are simultaneously credentialed in a health discipline that allows you to do so. *(Competence and Scope of Practice—5)*

2. You perform services only in areas for which you have "received education, training, supervised experience, or other study" that qualifies you for providing those services. *(Competence and Scope of Practice—1)*

3. You take steps to ensure that your personal biases, the boundaries of your competence, and the limitations of your training do not negatively impact the services you provide to your client. *(Personal and Interpersonal Boundaries—1)*

4. You understand the "limitations and subjective nature" of energy testing. *(The Healing Relationship—11)*

5. You engage each client in creating an appropriate plan of care, which may, as appropriate, include engaging other health-care professionals. *(The Healing Relationship—1)*

Your sense of alarm is the guiding perception in this situation. Keeping in mind that it is not unusual to come across energies in a new client that feel unfamiliar, you could begin by using all the energy assessment tools available to look for patterns that are consistent with an aggressive physical disorder (e.g., there are no figure eights in the area of concern, the spleen and/or kidney meridian cannot be made strong, pain in the related meridians or organs, and other physical symptoms reported by the client).

If you sill feel alarm after having investigated, it is appropriate and necessary to inform the person that you are concerned about energy irregularities and to make a referral to a physician or other health professional capable of making an appropriate diagnosis. You would not name the suspected diagnosis. That is outside your scope of practice. Using language such as "energy irregularities in the lower abdominal area" and "strong concern" and insisting that the appointment with the physician or other health professional be made before further sessions with you are scheduled are ways of conveying your sense of alarm.

Along with conveying your sense of alarm, it is equally important to convey that you do not *know* that something is seriously wrong, which, indeed, you do not. So you would need to establish a balance between conveying enough concern to motivate the person to get a proper diagnosis and not so much as to throw him or her into panic or undue worry. You will also want to word your recommendation so that if the test shows no serious illness, the person will still want to work with you (e.g., "I'm just puzzled by the energies. I don't know what they mean, but it would be irresponsible of me not to insist that you check it out medically.")

CASE VIGNETTE 8

You are extremely attracted to one of your clients, whom you have had three sessions with and are continuing to see weekly. You find yourself looking forward to this client's sessions and fantasizing about a personal relationship. What actions do you take in response to your feelings?

Thinking It Through

Relationships formed in energy healing sessions are built on a mutual understanding that the purpose of the relationship is to work toward the client's health goals through the use of energy healing techniques. Because this is an intimate process, and we are all human, feelings and fantasies that do not stay within those boundaries are not unnatural. The preponderance of experience from within the healing professions is, however, that when a practitioner's *behaviors* cross those boundaries, the healing relationship is compromised, the client is frequently harmed, and the sanctity of the healing setting as a safe haven is seriously threatened. For these reasons, the healing professions have developed numerous guidelines and mandates to keep professional relationships from leading to romantic or sexual involvements. Those in the "Ethics Code for Energy Healing Practitioners" include:

1. Dual relationships that are never acceptable are ones in which a practitioner develops any kind of romantic or sexual relationship with any client while energy healing services are being provided. *(Personal and Interpersonal Boundaries—17)*

2. You do not engage in sexual relations with a former client for at least a year after termination of the client relationship, and only then after a good faith determination through appropriate consultation that there is no exploitation of the former client. *(Personal and Interpersonal Boundaries—18)*

3. You remain sensitive to differences in power between the practitioner and the client and do not exploit such differences during or after the professional relationship. *(Personal and Interpersonal Boundaries—10)*

4. You closely monitor your needs to be liked or admired as well as your sexual and romantic needs and seek feedback, guidance, consultation, and supervision from friends, colleagues, mentors, supervisors, or other professionals to keep these needs from interfering with your effectiveness in the services you provide. *(Personal Healing and Development—6)*

If romantic feelings or fantasies enter your relationship with a client, it is always a good time to look within. You may decide they are natural and innocent. But if you are having difficulty containing such feelings or fantasies, it is a time to examine deeply.

Before accepting the public trust of offering energy healing services within your community, you made a firm commitment to maintain professional boundaries with your clients and to maintain strong sexual/romantic boundaries in particular. What is occurring within you that is straining the limits of your professional commitments and threatening your entire professional life? What unmet personal needs are spilling into your professional relationships? How can you better meet them? What unresolved emotional issue is this client tapping into? Asking these questions can—often with the aid of a psychotherapist, supervisor, colleague, or close friend—ultimately serve your personal evolution.

At a minimum, when romantic/sexual feelings or fantasies about a client persist, your first step should be to inform a colleague and enter a formal or informal consultative relationship with your colleague about this case. Experience suggests that the mind, even of a sincere professional health-care provider, can powerfully rationalize inappropriate behavior when driven by romantic and/or sexual desire. Subjecting such a situation to supervision immediately is a step you should have decided in advance—by both ironclad rule and self-commitment—to take.

The consultant can also help you sort through the various dynamics that may be involved. Just as the hormones influencing romantic love are often the most intense during a relationship's early stages, emotions involving attraction and the obsession with involvement may have an elevated intensity at the beginning stages of a healing relationship. If the right chemistry between the two individuals is present, this may be true for both parties. Understanding that this is likely to transform itself for both within the first six sessions gives you a framework for your internal perspective as well as how you might respond to a client professing love for you. The consultant can help you gauge what is unfolding and how to channel that energy into the growth of a creative healing relationship.

Often, bringing in a consultant or supervisor will itself shift the energy for you. The power of being unambiguously watched by the entire profession, through the concerned eyes of one of its members, has a way of cooling ardor, as does the commitment it represents of placing professional ethics above personal impulse. Self-examination of the needs and/or unresolved emotional issues this client is triggering in you may also be personally illuminating. If you and your supervisor find that your feelings or fantasies are persistent and are interfering with your work with your client, referral to another practitioner should be considered. The "One-Year Rule" *(Personal and Interpersonal Boundaries—18)* is designed to ensure that terminating the professional relationship is not simply a gambit to move into a romantic or sexual relationship with the client. The profession treats these issues with the utmost seriousness.

Other Considerations. Although there are differences between a psychotherapy practice (where therapist-client emotional dynamics play a more critical role in the work) and a non-psychotherapy energy healing practice (where the energetic dynamics can still serve or impede the healing process), maintaining the sanctity of the practitioner-client relationship—a key ethic in psychotherapy—is also critical in an energy healing practice. If you deviate from the formal guidelines that suggest you keep strong boundaries between the professional and personal spheres, the burden of proof will be on you that you have kept the client's best interests as your highest priority, that you did not exploit the power differences in the relationship, that you are not using your practice as a source for romantic or sexual liaisons, and that you have not diminished the sanctity of the energy healing relationship.

A major difference between psychotherapy and a non-psychotherapy energy healing practice, however, is that there are different degrees of involvement that you may have with a person seeking energy healing services. If the person is taking a one-evening class that teaches a five-minute energy routine, a professional relationship has still been entered, but it is of a different order than if you are providing intense ongoing individual sessions for a serious health challenge. It is also of a different order of involvement if an attraction on the practitioner's part is recognized and a consultation process is initiated after the first session or two rather than allowing the attraction to simmer without being acknowledged or dealt with until three months into the relationship.

It would almost always be inappropriate for you to be the one who *initiates* discussion about your attraction, particularly without first having discussed it with a consultant, and in no case should you discuss that attraction in a manner that even remotely implies that a romantic relationship between you and your client or student is a possibility. An important part of your job description is to create and maintain a safe space for learning and healing, and that includes maintaining the sanctity of your practice as a setting where you are not open to finding a life partner or more casual romantic liaisons.

That said, ethical situations often involve the collision of opposing forces or priorities. Suppose in twenty-two years of practice, you have never crossed the boundary discussed here. Then a participant in a brief class or a client who is new to your practice brings up, with no prompting from you, an attraction toward you (and you are both free of other commitments), and you are also experiencing intense feelings and fantasies. What are your options?

Your first action is to acknowledge your client's feelings while still maintaining your professional boundaries and keeping your attraction and fantasies to yourself. If, for some rare reason, you feel particularly compelled to pursue a personal relationship with the person and you have had very little contact in the healing context, it would probably be defensible to terminate the brief professional relationship (having made sure the client has access to other professional resources for addressing the needs being presented). Even here, however, with the healing relationship having hardly been consummated, you are well advised to seek consultation before revealing your feelings to the client and, if you decide to allow the relationship to become a personal one, to create a period of no contact, a "cooling off period." This gives time for both the early attraction to settle and the influence of the initial professional relationship to dissipate. A period of three months would seem a minimum requirement under any circumstances, and longer if a substantial healing relationship has been established. The American Psychological Association mandates two years. The "Ethics Code for Energy Healing Practitioners" suggests at least a year. At that point, you can start afresh and on more equal ground.

Whatever your reasons, the wisdom of the profession is that moving from a professional to a personal or romantic relationship contains many more hazards than may be obvious, particularly to newly infatuated individuals, however sophisticated they may be in other circumstances.

CASE VIGNETTE 9

Your client is being treated by a physician who is prescribing medication that you believe is both unnecessary and an obstacle rather than an aid to recovery. What do you do?

Thinking It Through

Non-physician energy healing practitioners are not authorized to prescribe medication, nor do they have the training of medical doctors about medication. Yet you have reason to believe, from an energy perspective, that the medication is not serving and is, in fact, harming your client. Ethical guidelines for this situation include:

1. You do not diagnose or treat medical illness unless simultaneously credentialed in a health discipline that allows you to do so. *(Competence and Scope of Practice—5)*

2. You recognize the limitations and subjective nature of nontraditional ways of assessing the flow within a client's energy system. *(The Healing Relationship—11)*

3. You take steps to ensure that your personal biases, the boundaries of your competence, and the limitations of your training do not negatively impact your service to your client. *(Personal and Interpersonal Boundaries—1)*

4. You treat colleagues with dignity, respect, and courtesy. *(Personal and Interpersonal Boundaries—12)*

5. You respect your client's right of self-determination. *(General Principles—7)*

6. When working with clients receiving health services elsewhere, you discuss these issues with the client in order to minimize risk of confusion and conflict, consult with other service providers when appropriate, and proceed with caution and sensitivity in a spirit of respect and cooperation toward all parties involved. *(Informed Consent—3)*

It is not appropriate to challenge the doctor's authority. You would never simply tell your client the medication is incorrect. The doctor is a professional working within a scope of competence that goes beyond your scope of competence. You can, however, take on the role of health advocate, helping the client to think through appropriate questions, such as whether there are alternative medications that could be considered if there are problematic side effects, how the dosage was determined, and whether the doctor has had experience with using this medication at other dosages. Frequently, it turns out the doctor has given the most common drug and dosage and is willing to adjust the dosage or try a different medication when problems are reported.

Thus a step the client can take is to observe carefully and systematically the effects of the medication on the malady the medication was prescribed to alleviate as well as symptoms that did not exist prior to starting the medication. This is information that should be provided to the physician. If your suspicions about the medication are correct, this would add the support of the client's own observations. Without that, you are in a tenuous situation unless you have a relationship with the physician or the physician understands and respects energy assessment methods. If the physician does understand and respect the methods you are using, you can offer your observations as you would to any other colleague, being appropriately conservative about the certainty of your speculation (for instance, you cannot make definitive health-care determinations or recommendations based on energy testing alone).

If the physician is not open to receiving such information from you, you should be particularly cautious in the language you use. The bottom line is that you do not have medically recognized tests or means for determining the impact of the medication. You can, however, show the client the results of the energy test when the client is touching the medication and explain your understanding of its implications, with appropriate disclaimers about the lack of medical certainty and the importance of not discontinuing a medication without the physician's supervision. Then it is up to the client to decide what to do with that information.

If the client continues to take the medication, you can take steps to support his or her energy system to help the body accept and metabolize the medication and to minimize side effects.

CASE VIGNETTE 10

A woman who has discovered a lump on her breast does not want to have a biopsy. She comes to you and asks you to use energy testing and intuition to determine if it is malignant. What do you do?

Thinking It Through

Unless licensed to do so, an energy healing practitioner cannot diagnose. Therefore your client's primary request is outside your scope of practice. Yet some of the information your client is requesting is within your scope of practice and potentially useful. Relevant guidelines include:

1. You do not diagnose or treat illness unless simultaneously credentialed in a health discipline that allows you to do so. (*Competence and Scope of Practice—5*)

2. You recognize the limitations and subjective nature of nontraditional ways of assessing the flow within a client's energy system. (*The Healing Relationship—11*)

3. You provide information to prospective clients about the limitations of your training regarding issues such as the diagnosis and treatment of

illness, possible side effects, and the fact that energy medicine is considered an unconventional approach to health care. *(Competence and Scope of Practice—2)*

4. You avoid unrealistic or unclear commitments. *(General Principles—5)*

5. You utilize an informed consent form to provide clear information to prospective clients about the nature of your services. *(Informed Consent—1)*

6. You exercise the right to refuse to accept into your care any person seeking services when you judge this not to be in the best interests of the client. *(Healing Relationship—7)*

Your prospective client's desire to rely on energy tests and on your intuition to determine if the lump on her breast is malignant assumes these are reliable enough sources of information to stake her life on them. Do you have solid grounds to be certain this is a valid assumption? If not, you can, with absolute conviction, discuss the problems involved in her desired course of action. Exploring with respect her concerns, beliefs, expectations, fears, and goals around this situation would be useful for deeply understanding her position. But if it is the case that the biopsy, while invasive, is in your best judgment the only way to ensure early treatment if the lump is malignant, possibly saving the woman's life, then this would also set the context for that discussion.

Of course, there are many circumstances in which an energetic assessment of the woman's breast, along with energy sessions that attempt to shift abnormal energies, may be appropriate and desirable. But if this means entering into complicity with the woman's hope that energy tests and intuition are as decisive as a biopsy, you are ethically obligated to resolve this issue before offering your services. Otherwise, you are giving the woman cause to continue to assume that the information you provide will be as reliable as a proper medical diagnosis, a step you should not take lightly. This is not a situation in which respecting a client's right to self-determination means that you would automatically comply with her request. If it is, in fact, clear to you that providing the requested information is going to lead to an interpretation of that information that is not properly informed or that will be skewed by wishful thinking, you are obligated to address the woman's inaccurate assumptions in advance.

Another assumption in her initial request that you should identify and challenge if you do work with her is the fundamental but false notion that an energy test can determine if a lump is malignant. Energy testing is designed to determine if the energy is flowing optimally through a specific meridian. That is the extent of it. See the discussion "What You Can't Energy Test" in *Energy Medicine* by Donna Eden with David Feinstein (rev. ed., 2008; pp. 64–65) for further guidance on this key issue in making assessments.

CASE VIGNETTE 11

Your client's physician wants her to stop seeing you because the physician believes that energy healing is quackery and might even do his patient harm. Meanwhile, the patient has not been able to find scientific evidence that energy healing is a legitimate treatment approach and is inclined to follow the physician's advice. But you believe your sessions with the client are just starting to have an impact and that terminating them would constitute a missed opportunity. What do you do?

Thinking It Through

You are not licensed to advise a client about diagnosis or treatment. The physician is. Yet you are using a complementary method that is gaining increasing recognition as a viable approach to health care, though a state license for using this approach is not yet available. Most important, you have reason to believe that your services are benefiting your client's health in ways the client does not yet recognize. Relevant guidelines include:

1. You may attempt to encourage, but you do not attempt to pressure or coerce a client into any action or belief, even if you anticipate such action or belief would serve the best interests of the client. *(Healing Relationship—3)*

2. You discuss these issues with the client in order to minimize the risk of confusion and conflict, consult with other service providers when appropriate, and proceed with caution and sensitivity in a spirit of respect and cooperation with all parties involved. *(Informed Consent—3)*

3. You encourage hope and convey confidence in energy healing methods without overstating the power of the methods. *(Healing Relationship—5)*

4. You use an informed consent form to provide clear information about your practice. *(Informed Consent—1)*

5. You reevaluate expectations throughout the professional relationship. *(The Healing Relationship—5)*

6. You do not become overly attached to the outcome of the services you provide. *(The Healing Relationship—6)*

7. You treat colleagues with dignity, respect, and courtesy. *(Personal and Interpersonal Boundaries—12)*

Enter the discussion with full respect for the client's ultimate decision. Stay on alert to avoid any subtle coercion on your part. At the same time, be willing to provide all the information available so that your client's decision, whether to stop or to continue working with you, is as well informed as possible.

It is appropriate for you to explain in detail your assessment of your client's energies, the choices you have made, the results you have seen, the results you anticipate with further sessions, and the probable impact of these results on your client's overall well-being. You can also encourage your client to reflect upon the sessions with questions such as: "What were your initial complaints and expectations?" "What effects did you observe?" "How do you understand what is occurring in the sessions?"

It is also appropriate to offer additional information about the approach you are using. A published, peer-reviewed, professional paper that provides an overview of the history, uses, mechanisms, and evidence for energy medicine can be found at *www.EnergyMedicinePrinciples.com*. A less formal overview of the field was written by Christiane Northrup, MD, as the foreword to Donna Eden's book, *Energy Medicine for Women*, available as a free download from *www.EnergyMedicineForWomen.com*. The "Energy Medicine Fact Sheet" in the *Toolkit for Energy Healing Practitioners* (*http://toolkit.innersource.net*) links to various energy medicine research sites. These could, as appropriate, be made available to your client and to the physician. Other energy healing books and articles you have found useful might also be used as sources of information you could offer.

Along with offering this information, you could offer to contact the physician to discuss and inform. You would, of course, need a signed release from your client. Although it is not your place to question your client's choice of physician, if you have a list of local physicians who collaborate with complementary health practitioners, there may be a place in the dialogue—such as if your client asks if there are local doctors who make referrals to you—where you would provide that information.

But in this entire process of providing information, keep in mind that energy healing isn't for everyone, explore your attachments to the outcome of the discussion, and "release" your client to make the best choice for her or himself at this time.

Additional Considerations. Terminating a professional relationship involves a number of subtle issues. Though it is appropriate to invite a client to discuss the reasons for deciding to stop seeing you, this may evoke feelings of rejection or defensiveness in you, and it is your responsibility to monitor them. In the end, this is the client's choice and, while you can explore the reasons behind the choice, your place is to accept the choice respectfully. In no instance should a client be made to feel guilty for choosing to leave a professional relationship.

In some relatively rare situations, a client's announcement that it is time to end the relationship is, at a deeper emotional level, a test of your loyalty or level of engagement. This can be addressed directly. The bottom line is that it is the person's right to leave, even while you affirm that the door is open should he or she wish to return.

In a situation in which you need to end the relationship, it is important to discuss with the client the timeline and process that would be the most constructive. This honors the relationship that you have had and recognizes that abrupt termination, even of a relationship that is no longer workable, for whatever reasons, may not be in the client's best interest. Tapering off the visits, or scheduling a final visit a month or two down the road may also allow appropriate closure of a long and deep healing relationship that has run its positive course.

CASE VIGNETTE 12

You have just completed a powerful regression session and you learn that the client has a Rolfing session scheduled that evening. You are concerned that the Rolfing might prevent an integration of the regression

work and might even be harmful. Can you ask a client to reschedule a session with another practitioner?

Thinking It Through

Sometimes a powerful session needs time for integration and too quickly engaging in an intensive form of therapy may be contraindicated. Guidelines to consider include:

1. You hold as your highest priority the health and welfare of your client. *(General Principles—1)*

2. Your obligation is to make sure clients understand and agree to the specifics of the work before commencing energy healing services. *(Informed Consent—2)*

3. You consider the health-care issue and the client's welfare and discuss them in order to minimize the risk of confusion and conflict and proceed with caution in a spirit of respect and cooperation with all parties involved. *(Informed Consent—3)*

4. You engage the client in identifying goals for the services being sought and mutually create a plan of care, which may also include other health-care professionals. *(The Healing Relationship—1)*

5. You clarify professional roles and obligations and seek to manage conflicts of interest. *(Personal and Interpersonal Boundaries—2)*

If your sense after the regression session is that the Rolfing session might be detrimental to your client, based on the work that was just completed, you are obligated, for the client's welfare, to express this and, with your client, to think through possible courses of action. While you must respect that it is ultimately the client's choice, postponing the Rolfing session might be the desired outcome. Offering to contact the Rolfing practitioner to explain the situation is one possible means toward that outcome. Some regression work within the context of Eden Energy Medicine involves planned, extended sessions, and guidelines covering situations such as this are to be conveyed to the client in advance. If you were negligent in making it clear that another intensive body-oriented session was contraindicated, you might take responsibility for the financial consequences of canceling the session. This is not to suggest that you should put yourself into this position, but on the contrary, that your communications should be so clear and direct as to prevent this kind of situation.

CASE VIGNETTE 13

You are working with your client's neurolymphatic points. Your client is clearly in considerable discomfort. How do you determine if you are applying too much pressure? If you determine the pressure is therapeutic, do you ignore the client's discomfort?

Thinking It Through

Neurolymphatic massage is among the most subjectively invasive procedures within energy healing. Relevant guidelines include:

1. Energy healing shall always be administered in a caring, considerate manner, with respect for the client's preferences and capacities. You inform your client of the purpose of any invasive procedures and offer an explicit choice about whether to proceed or to have alternative methods applied. If the choice is to proceed, agreement is reached in advance how the client will communicate to you the desire to stop the procedure. You will immediately respect this signal and halt the procedure. *(The Healing Relationship—12)*

2. You are sensitive to a client's feelings about being touched and discuss those feelings as appropriate. *(The Healing Relationship—13)*

3. You recognize that clear, compassionate communication is integral to providing the highest level of service possible and you act accordingly. *(Personal and Interpersonal Boundaries—3)*

If you use a procedure that the client is likely to find painful, such as placing pressure on a neurolymphatic point, you inform the client about the procedure and its purpose in advance and offer an explicit choice about whether to proceed or to have alternative methods applied. You also establish in advance how your client will let you know if he or she wants you to stop.

As with any invasive procedure, you are sensitive to the way it may evoke earlier experiences of physical pain or abuse and discuss and calibrate as appropriate.

While pain on a neurolymphatic point often indicates congested energy, you must check to be certain that the pain is not being caused by an injury or other medical condition. It is your responsibility to ensure that the neurolymphatic work will not bruise or in any other way cause physical damage. Be alert to a stoicism in certain clients who might not admit to discomfort they nonetheless do not wish to tolerate.

Even after this education and preparation, you should not ignore your client's discomfort but, along with supportive and reassuring comments, recheck that he or she is okay with the current level of discomfort. Clients always have the final say in setting the pace and intensity of energy healing work.

CASE VIGNETTE 14

You are a female working with a male client's neurolymphatic points and have come to the pubic bone. His penis is covering some of the points. What do you do?

Thinking It Through

In work that involves touching another person's body, you may encounter various types of awkward or sensitive situations. Relevant guidelines include:

1. You are sensitive to a client's feelings about being touched and discuss those feelings as appropriate. If a procedure requires making contact or putting pressure in the area of a client's genitals, breasts, buttocks, navel, or throat, as the practitioner you are particularly alert to the client's sensitivities and offer alternative methods if appropriate, such as asking clients to use their own hands in making the direct contact. *(The Healing Relationship—13)*

2. Clients shall be informed in advance about the purpose of any invasive procedures and given an explicit choice about whether to proceed or to have alternative methods applied. *(The Healing Relationship—12)*

3. You do not engage in sexual harassment. Sexual harassment includes conduct that is sexual in nature, that occurs in connection with your professional role or activities, and that is: (1) unwelcome, offensive, or

creates an objectionable interpersonal atmosphere and the practitioner has been informed of this; (2) is sufficiently severe or intense to be considered abusive to a reasonable person in the same context; or (3) is unnecessarily or inappropriately provocative under the guise of evaluating a health concern or providing services. *(Personal and Interpersonal Boundaries—20)*

Straightforward communication about the neurolymphatics and how you work with them will prevent many potential problems or misunderstandings. Also, the client can easily be instructed to work with the points on his pubic bone or to make direct contact with his own hand so that you are placing the pressure on his hand instead of his pubic bone. If you are going to apply the pressure directly, letting him know that you need access to his pubic bone can be done in a straightforward manner. You are mindful to communicate in such a way that it is clear to your client that this touch is not intended to be construed as sexual in any way and that any touch that the client tells you is uncomfortable will immediately be ceased.

CASE VIGNETTE 15

A man who has heard of your ability to sense energies asks you to assess whether he needs a colonoscopy, a procedure that was routinely recommended because he has just turned fifty. You have a very clear perception from sensing his energies, as well as from energy testing, that he does not require the procedure. What do you do?

Thinking It Through

Although here you are dealing with a different medical condition from that of vignette 10, the same principles apply.

CASE VIGNETTE 16

A man consults you after his wife is diagnosed with lung cancer. He had been a smoker for the thirty years of their marriage and she had complained about this for thirty years. He gave up smoking immediately after her diagnosis, and his guilt is enormous. The wife is interested only

in a conventional medical approach. He wants to pursue every possible avenue to help her and has heard that energy healing can be done on a remote basis. You ask for her consent, but he begs you to "just do it" because she already has too much on her mind and introducing her to such a strange concept might overwhelm her. Can you do the healings for her without her explicit permission?

Thinking It Through

Einstein described the nonlocal connections (entanglement) of quantum physics as "spooky action at a distance," and this seems to describe surrogate healing as well. Strong scientific evidence demonstrating the impact of thought and intention on the physical world is available to anyone who cares to look (see, for instance, Dean Radin's *Entangled Minds*). The husband believes you can use surrogate healing to help his wife, noninvasively and without adding to her stress or concerns. The wife, however, is not your client, has not been consulted about this plan, and has expressed her desire to use only conventional medicine. Relevant guidelines include:

1. You do not diagnose or treat illness unless you are simultaneously credentialed in a health discipline that allows you to do so. (*Competence and Scope of Practice—5*)

2. You respect the rights of individuals to privacy, confidentiality, and self-determination. (*General Principles—7*)

3. You obtain explicit or clearly implied permission prior to engaging in "distant" or "remote" or "surrogate" or "nonlocal" assessment or healing. (*Personal and Interpersonal Boundaries—11*)

4. You know your limitations and set boundaries accordingly with those you serve, your colleagues, and the larger community. (*Personal Healing and Development—4*)

5. You encourage hope in energy healing methods without overstating their power or fostering guilt. (*The Healing Relationship—4*)

6. You may attempt to encourage, but you do not attempt to pressure or coerce a client into any action or belief, even if you consider that such act or belief would serve the best interests of the client. (*The Healing Relationship—3*)

The wife's informed consent is as much a necessity in a distant healing situation as it would be in the office. There may be no such restriction about praying for someone, but distant healing is generally understood as being quite different from prayer, and attempting to heal the wife without her consent would be an invasion of her boundaries.

At the same time that you are turning down the husband's request, you can use the situation to educate him about his most viable options in supporting his wife. You might start by acknowledging his caring and his desire to help his wife and then help him gain a better understanding about boundaries. Just as secondhand smoke invades the lungs of those nearby, his more benevolent request still involves boundary issues. You might explain to him how it serves his wife's best interests if he does everything he can do to support her right to be in control of her care and treatment.

Since he has consulted you, you may offer to help him to keep his energies balanced as he engages the challenges of his wife's illness, while pointing out that his staying healthy and vibrant will benefit his wife as well, and that his benefit from energy healing would be one of the best possible advertisements for encouraging his wife to give it a try. You might also use techniques for emotional balancing for addressing his fears, sorrow, and guilt.

Regarding his wife's health care, you can explain to him how energy healing can be used in conjunction with conventional medicine, and you can provide him with information that he can share with his wife *when she is ready*. You can offer to make an appointment with her and/or her doctor to discuss how energy healing might help her without interfering in planned conventional treatments, if and when that is appropriate.

CASE VIGNETTE 17

You have been developing your ability in remote viewing and surrogate healing. You have a session with a young man in a few hours and have been thinking about his case. Can you "tune in" to him as you consider how you can best serve him?

Thinking It Through

The wording of this question implies that your skills in remote viewing are well developed. The young man is seeking your help. You want to help him.

But to the extent that your remote viewing capacities are well developed, you also have the tools to invade his privacy. Relevant guidelines include:

1. You respect your client's rights to privacy, confidentiality, and self-determination. *(General Principles—7)*

2. You obtain explicit or clearly implied permission prior to engaging in "distant," "remote," "surrogate," or "nonlocal" assessment or healing. *(Personal and Interpersonal Boundaries—11)* You perform such services only after having carefully considered the issues described in the "Handout Bank" article about distance healing (*www.HandoutBank. org*).

3. You provide services only in areas in which you have received education, training, supervised experience, or other study that qualifies you for providing those services. *(Competence and Scope of Practice—1)*

4. You are sensitive to differences in power between the practitioner and the client and do not exploit such differences. *(Personal and Interpersonal Boundaries—10)*

A number of boundary issues are involved in this case. On the safe side of the boundary, few people would object to one person sending another person good wishes or good energies. Praying for someone else's health or well-being is not usually considered a boundary violation, even by those not inclined toward prayer. Clearing your mind prior to a session, reviewing the previous session, and letting your intuition guide you about the upcoming session is certainly appropriate. But in this case, you have been developing your capacity for remote viewing. This may cross over to the other side of the boundary.

The first ethical issue here is permission. A healer with remote viewing capacities is required, according to energy healing ethics, to gain explicit permission before engaging in remote viewing or surrogate healing activities. When the individual is not able to provide that permission, such as if the person is an infant or is in a coma, permission from the legal guardian or custodian must be obtained.

There is, however, also a distinction between a remote viewing/surrogate healing session and other ways of caring about a person from a distance. When thinking about a client, it may be hard to distinguish your thoughts and intuition from channeled or "nonlocal" information.

Knowledge may come to you without your intending to evoke nonlocal information. Intention is the key here. If you focus on a person with the intent of remote viewing or surrogate healing, permission is required.

CASE VIGNETTE 18

Your client has brought in a medication that has just been prescribed and wants you to energy test it. You find that it tests weak. How do you explain this finding to your client?

Thinking It Through

Many of the principles identified in vignette 9 also apply here.

The difference is that in this situation the client has not yet taken the medication and is explicitly asking you to assess its energetic impact before he or she takes it. In explaining the significance of the energy test, appropriate disclaimers are critical. You are not licensed or trained in the indications and contraindications regarding medication. Information gained from energy tests should only be used in the context of other sources of information. Energy testing is not infallible, and its efficacy is not firmly established by scientific research. Your own or the client's beliefs or fears may, in fact, have impacted the energy test. The medication might be necessary and effective, yet the test may reveal an energetic reaction that masks these benefits. The energetic reaction might, in fact, provide a clue as to how energy work can be used to make your client's body more receptive to the benefits of the medication. Checking the medication against each meridian and balancing meridians that go into reaction while in the energy field of the medication can help the body to better utilize the medication.

On the other hand, the medication may be truly harmful or the prescribed dosage may not be right for your client. If balancing the affected meridians will not hold, this may be a clue. If testing the medication against the meridian or other energy system that governs the physical condition the medication is intended to help disrupts that energy system, this may also be a clue. Though all the disclaimers listed previously still apply, this additional information may also be ethically revealed to the client.

Your job is to be certain that your client understands what is and what is not within your scope of practice (advising about whether or not to take the medication is outside your scope of practice; educating your client about how to assess the likely energetic impact of a substance on specific meridians is within your scope of practice), and to provide balanced information that promotes an informed decision. If the client does decide against the medication, you are obligated to insist that the client consult and inform the physician before taking that action. Along with the need for you to respect the physician's professional role in the case, abrupt discontinuation of some medications can be harmful. You should let the client know you are available to talk with the physician and should be prepared to explain that you did *not* advise the client to stop the medication, as well as exactly what you did do and why.

CASE VIGNETTE 19

Your client is having terrible PMS. You have several herbal remedies and you energy test them, showing that one in particular tests very strong. Do you recommend that she go to the health food store and purchase it? Do you energy test for a product that you, yourself, sell?

Thinking It Through

The combination of herbal remedies and hands-on energy healing techniques can be potent and beneficial. Several guidelines apply:

1. You respect the rights of individuals to self-determination. *(General Principles—7)*

2. You may attempt to encourage, but you do not attempt to pressure or coerce a client into any action or belief, even if you consider that such act or belief would serve the best interests of the client. *(The Healing Relationship—3)*

3. You recognize the pitfalls of being overly attached to the outcomes of the work you provide. *(The Healing Relationship—6)*

4. You are particularly cautious about energy testing potential customers on products you are selling. *(The Healing Relationship—11)*

5. You may recommend nutritional supplements, technological devices, or other healing aids only when you have adequate and appropriate knowledge to make such recommendations responsibly. *(The Healing Relationship—17)*

6. You do your best to ensure that your personal biases, the boundaries of your competence, and the limitations of your training do not negatively impact the services you provide to your clients. *(Personal and Interpersonal Boundaries—1)*

The wording of the question suggests that you have herbs in your office that you are recommending, or not, based in part on energy testing. The cautions about the reliability of energy testing for substances, discussed in the previous vignette, apply to herbs as well as to medications. If you are recommending herbs, you are required to have sufficient training to make those recommendations responsibly, including knowledge about the research supporting claims regarding the herb's benefits, how to select from many possibilities the substance that is most appropriate for your client, potential side effects, and possible dangerous interactions between the herb and any medications the client is taking.

Assuming you have the proper training, are making your recommendations within the framework of local and state statutes, and are including appropriate disclaimers, the conflict of interest issue remains if you are selling the product you are recommending. To provide health-care services while also selling the products you are recommending puts you in a dual relationship with your clients. Though many health-care practitioners do indeed sell products they believe will be beneficial for their clients, you are well advised to avoid a situation that would appear to be a conflict to outside observers, and that might indeed compromise your objectivity in making recommendations. Backing your recommendations with energy testing, which can be influenced in conflict-of-interest situations, is particularly suspect.

The cleanest arrangement is to provide contact information for vendors of the products you are recommending, vendors with whom you have no financial involvement. If the nature of your practice is such that it is important for the client to have immediate access to herbal remedies that you recommend, one way you could carry such products and minimize the conflict of interest is to sell them at your cost. Avoiding the appearance of impropriety, as well as doing all in your power to support objectivity in your recommendations, is of central importance here.

CASE VIGNETTE 20

Your client comes in reporting that she is very unhappy with the treatment she has been receiving from you. She has been doing everything you have recommended and her original condition has not improved after five sessions. The two of you are unable to come to an understanding. The client wants a refund and an apology. You feel you have been following protocol, are puzzled by the lack of response, and do not know the next step. What do you do?

Thinking It Through

Your services, delivered to the best of your ability, have not led to the desired outcomes and you are not sure of the reasons or of how to proceed in a manner that would lead to a better outcome. Your client wants not only to discontinue her work with you, but she is also asking for a refund and an apology. Relevant guidelines include:

1. You engage each client in identifying goals for the services being sought and mutually create an appropriate plan of care. *(The Healing Relationship—1)*

2. You may attempt to encourage, but you do not attempt to pressure or coerce a client into any action or belief, even if you consider that such act or belief would serve the best interests of the client. *(The Healing Relationship—3)*

3. Though it is appropriate to encourage hope and convey confidence in energy healing methods, you do so without overstating the power of the methods or implying that a method that has helped some people with a particular health issue will help all people with that issue. You also proceed with a sensitivity to avoid fostering guilt in clients who are not responding as hoped. *(The Healing Relationship—4)*

4. You elicit each client's expectations about energy healing and the client's goals in using it, restating them to the client for clarity and agreement, and discussing any unrealistic expectations, before providing services. Expectations are reevaluated throughout the professional relationship at times you deem appropriate or at any time at the client's request. *(The Healing Relationship—5)*

5. You recognize the pitfalls of being overly attached to the outcomes of the services you provide. "Trying too hard," micromanaging a client, or becoming overly invested may have a paradoxical effect. *(The Healing Relationship—6)*

6. You terminate a client relationship when it becomes reasonably clear that the client no longer needs or is no longer benefiting from the continued service. *(The Healing Relationship—18)*

7. If you reach an interpersonal impasse with a client or an impasse in the healing services you are providing, you may seek supervision, suggest bringing a consultant into a session, refer the client to another practitioner, or suggest terminating the services. *(The Healing Relationship—19)*

Your client has every right to discontinue services at any point. If you have indeed followed protocol and provided informed consent, you are not legally or ethically required to provide a refund. The contract is payment for time providing professional services. Outcome is not guaranteed.

However, this person came to you in good faith and did not receive the hoped-for benefits. You have any number of choices in how to handle the situation. You may choose to do more than you are legally or ethically required to do out of your care for the client, your pride in your work and in your reputation, and/or a desire to resolve any ill will. You could indeed apologize for, or at least acknowledge, the time and expense that did not lead to the desired outcome and make whatever restitution you feel is appropriate. You could articulate your puzzlement and make a referral to someone who you feel might be able to penetrate the mystery. You could refund all or a portion of your fee. You could offer a free session in which you bring in an advanced energy healing practitioner as a consultant (or arrange a Skype consultation of a live session). Though this would require an investment on your part, the fact that you do not know what is interfering with the client's progress might make it a very good investment, both for your own professional education (and reputation) and for the client's welfare, as well as an investment in possibly getting over a hurdle and being able to continue to work productively with the client.

CASE VIGNETTE 21

You receive an e-mail from someone in another region asking you for advice on how to use energy healing with a specific condition. The person has read Donna Eden's book *Energy Medicine,* **watched several DVDs, is trying to self-treat, and found you on a Web listing of energy healing practitioners. What are your responsibilities? Must you respond at all? If so, how soon?**

Thinking It Through

Even though the e-mail was unsolicited, your e-mail address is being made available because you are offering professional services, and a professional response within a reasonable time period is called for. Relevant guidelines include:

1. You engage each client in mutually creating an appropriate plan of care, including enlisting other health-care professionals. *(The Healing Relationship—1)*

2. You assist others in developing informed judgments concerning the role of energy healing in choices that impact their health and optimal functioning. *(Public Statements—1)*

3. Though it is appropriate to encourage hope and to convey confidence in energy healing methods, you do so without overstating the power of the methods or implying that a method that has helped some people with a particular health issue will help all people with that issue. *(The Healing Relationship—4)*

The professional response required of you can take many forms, depending in part on the nature of the request and the amount of time you are willing to provide before an actual paid relationship is established. You could simply provide a somewhat stock answer to the person's question. You could answer the question and send the person an electronic copy of "A Beginner's Guide to Energy Medicine" (from the *Toolkit for Energy Healing Practitioners, http://toolkit.innersource.net*) as background to your answer. You could tell the person about energy healing practitioners and classes that may be available locally. You could offer, if the situation warrants, to establish a paid telephone, e-mail, or Skype consultation relationship. You could explain, if the situation dictates, that without seeing the person, you cannot properly assess the energies, and make a referral to a local practitioner or explain how to locate a qualified local practitioner.

CASE VIGNETTE 22

Your client has a growth that you believe may be malignant. Your client refuses to get a medical diagnosis. You are deeply concerned and feel the situation is urgent. You plead and cajole. Your client still refuses. You know your client's doctor's name and your client's spouse. What are your responsibilities?

Thinking It Through

You suspect a medical condition that you are unable to diagnose definitively and your client refuses to obtain a proper medical diagnosis. Though your client is coming to you for an unrelated condition, you are still offering services as a health-care provider. Relevant guidelines include:

1. Your client is the only person who has the right to determine who has access to information about the energy healing services he or she has received from you. *(Confidentiality—1)*

2. You do not diagnose or treat illness unless you are simultaneously credentialed in a health discipline that allows you to do so. *(Competence and Scope of Practice—5)*

3. You respect the rights of individuals to self-determination. *(General Principles—7)*

4. You may attempt to encourage, but you do not attempt to pressure or coerce a client into any action or belief, even if you consider that such act or belief would serve the best interests of the client. *(The Healing Relationship—3)*

5. You recognize the pitfalls of being overly attached to the outcomes of the services you provide. "Trying too hard" may have a paradoxical effect. *(The Healing Relationship—6)*

6. You recognize the limitations and subjective nature of nontraditional ways of assessing the flow within a client's energy system. *(The Healing Relationship—11)*

7. If conflicts occur regarding your ethical obligations (such as when your commitment to your client's welfare comes into conflict with confidentiality requirements and other considerations), you attempt to resolve these conflicts in a responsible fashion that avoids or minimizes harm. *(The Healing Relationship—15)*

8. Because energy healing can open issues that are delicate, you are prepared to articulate these issues when they emerge and discuss them in a frank, professional, and respectful manner, while at the same time acknowledging the client's right not to discuss the issue. *(Personal and Interpersonal Boundaries—4)*

You want to ensure that your client's health is not compromised by the ignoring of available warning signs. Yet the majority of the guidelines suggest that you must honor the client's choices as well as the client's confidentiality. You can break confidentiality when there is "clear and imminent danger," but, while you may suspect the worst, this situation does not meet that criterion. So contacting the client's physician or spouse without the client's permission would violate confidentiality.

If you have been adamant about your recommendation for a medical diagnosis, you could then leave it in the client's hands. You are instructed to articulate delicate issues having to do with the client's welfare, but you are also instructed not to be coercive. Your largest leverage would be to make it a condition for continuing to work together that the client obtain a medical diagnosis. Though this borders on being coercive rather than honoring the client's choice, you may find that it is the only route you can take in good conscience, explaining to the client that the work you are doing on the digestive difficulties (or whatever has brought the person to see you) will have little ultimate value if it contributes to the client not receiving potentially lifesaving treatment.

CASE VIGNETTE 23

You wake up with a bad stomachache and a mild temperature. You have five clients scheduled this day, including one who has traveled a considerable distance to see you. What do you do?

Thinking It Through

You *could* push through your stomach discomfort and keep your appointments, and you feel a strong responsibility to your clients. Should you? Relevant guidelines include:

1. You monitor the effects of your physical health on your ability to help those with whom you work. *(Personal Healing and Development—2)*

2. You provide a safe environment for your services that is conducive to healing. *(The Healing Relationship—9)*

3. You acknowledge a special responsibility to take steps to keep your own energy systems strong and resilient. *(Personal and Interpersonal Boundaries—7)*

4. If you are unable to offer services due to illness, you cancel or postpone the activity until the limiting factors have been resolved. *(Personal and Interpersonal Boundaries—8)*

The guidelines are clear. You should *not* be providing healing services when you are ill or when your "energetic integrity" is compromised.

You would model appropriate self-care by canceling your appointments for the day. If there is a local practitioner who is able to see those whose needs are most urgent or the one who traveled a distance, you may try to arrange this.

The gray area is that a stomachache and a mild temperature can be turned around quite rapidly by the self-application of energy work. While canceling the appointments in order to courteously give your clients as much notice as possible, you might keep open the possibility of providing a session or two later in the day, with the clear understanding that if you are still not feeling restored, you will have to let them know you are not available.

CASE VIGNETTE 24

You know that one of the faculty members has been telling a friend who is also a student in an energy healing certification program what is going to be covered on the graduation exam. What do you do with this information? What do you do when you know another energy healing practitioner has committed an ethical violation?

Thinking It Through

Though only two people are directly involved in the situation, their unethical actions reverberate into the larger community. You recognize that revealing to a student the content of the graduation exam is a direct violation of the faculty member's professional responsibilities, but you are unsure of what steps you are obligated to take. Relevant guidelines include:

1. If you believe there may have been an ethical violation by another energy healing practitioner, you attempt to resolve the issue by bringing it to the attention of that individual if an informal resolution appears possible and appropriate. If the issue is not or cannot be adequately resolved in that fashion, you take further action appropriate to the circumstances. Such action might include informing the relevant ethics committee of the situation. *(The Resolution of Ethical Issues—1, 2)*

2. You treat your colleague with dignity, respect, and courtesy. *(Personal and Interpersonal Boundaries—12)*

Your first step is made clear by the "Ethics Code for Energy Healing Practitioners." You are expected to approach the faculty member in question and, using respectful, clear communication, address the issue. You are stepping forward not just with your personal concerns, but also as a member of the energy healing community who is obligated to take action upon learning that an ethical rule may have been violated. Depending on your source, you may need first to determine whether the information you have is accurate. If it is accurate, you need to hear the faculty member's side of the story. If a serious breach of ethics has occurred, and there is no reasonable remedy, you must inform the ethics committee. A caveat is if you are a student, which means there is a power difference between you and the faculty member. In that case, you could bring your concern to another faculty member and ask that person to intervene.

CASE VIGNETTE 25

You intuitively sense that a particular certified practitioner is deeply troubled and that this is compromising the person's work. While you

have no direct information that the practitioner is not doing a good job, another member of the community heatedly mentions a concern about this same practitioner. Do you share your intuitive hit?

Thinking It Through

This is a very delicate situation in which the lines between fact and impression, sharing and gossip, are very thin. Relevant guidelines include:

1. You monitor your needs to be liked, to be admired, to achieve status, and to exercise power. *(Personal Healing and Development—6)*

2. You recognize that clear, compassionate communication is integral to providing the highest level of service possible and act accordingly. *(Personal and Interpersonal Boundaries—3)*

3. You treat colleagues with dignity, respect, and courtesy; resist gossip; and talk about colleagues in respectful ways. *(Personal and Interpersonal Boundaries—12)*

4. If you believe there may have been an ethical violation by another energy healing practitioner, you attempt to resolve the issue by bringing it to the attention of that individual if an informal resolution appears possible and appropriate. If the issue is not adequately resolved through these informal steps, you take further action appropriate to the circumstances. Such action might include informing the relevant ethics committee about the situation. *(The Resolution of Ethical Issues—1, 2)*

Although it might be tempting to use this situation as an opportunity to vent your feelings, these feelings should instead be shared with the practitioner in question. You can do this in a highly respectful and caring way, letting the person know you have some intuitive concerns and perhaps that you have heard some gossip, but you do not have other kinds of evidence. Since, however, your concerns relate to the colleague's professional activities, you thought it appropriate to share them and offer support. Similarly, in listening to your other colleague speaking about the person, it is fine to register what is being said, but your responses should be oriented toward having the person share these concerns directly with the practitioner. If the situation develops so that the concerns cannot be resolved in this way—such as if the person refuses to have the conversation or ignores the feedback—and if substantive evidence emerges, the ethics committee of your professional association is there to investigate further if appropriate.

CASE VIGNETTE 26

At this point (continuing #25), a student in one of your classes asks if you recommend that he schedule a session with the practitioner in question. You have no direct knowledge that the practitioner is not providing good services. How do you respond?

Thinking It Through

You are feeling concerns about an energy healing practitioner, though you have no hard evidence. At this point, you are asked by one of your students if you recommend the very same practitioner. Guidelines that might be relevant in this case are:

1. You hold as the highest priority in your professional activities the health and welfare of your clients and students. *(General Principles—1)*

2. You promote accuracy, honesty, and truthfulness in your communications. *(General Principles—4)*

3. You treat colleagues with dignity, respect, and courtesy; resist gossip; and talk about colleagues in respectful ways. *(Personal and Interpersonal Boundaries—12)*

4. When you believe there may have been an ethical violation by another energy healing practitioner, you attempt to resolve the issue by bringing it to the attention of that individual in an informal resolution if that appears possible and appropriate. *(The Resolution of Ethical Issues—1)*

5. You show respect for various personalities, rhythms, representational styles, educational levels, and backgrounds; do not falsely impugn the reputation of your colleagues; and do not file or encourage the filing of ethics complaints that are made with disregard for facts that would disprove the allegation. *(The Resolution of Ethical Issues—5)*

This is delicate and subjective. As you examine your primary responsibility in the situation, it will become clear that it is your first priority to serve the best interests of the student, with a focus on helping him find a suitable practitioner.

Though you cannot, of course, present concerns that have no foundation in facts, ignoring your intuitive sense and wholeheartedly endorsing the practitioner would not be in full integrity either.

The situation catches you in mid-thought. You are feeling your concerns but have not yet had a chance to present them to the practitioner. Several possible courses of action are open to you. If you wish to talk first with the practitioner, you could tell the student that you would like a bit of time to think about whom you would recommend. Or you could tell the student that you do not have the kind of information you would need to be able to advise for or against consulting the practitioner. You could also coach the student on how to do a telephone or e-mail interview with a practitioner prior to setting up a session to see if it feels like a fit, with a focus on empowering the student to get the best services possible.

You could also let your student know that you have no direct experience with this practitioner but that you do highly recommend someone whose work you know quite intimately. Also, keep in mind that some clients will receive much more benefit from a given practitioner than others and that it would be wise for your student to interview several potential practitioners.

Case Vignette 27

You are present when several of your energy healing colleagues are discussing their concerns about the treatment choices a specific practitioner has been making. To your knowledge, these concerns, though they seem legitimate to you, have not been shared with the practitioner. Do you immediately turn the person in to the appropriate ethics committee or send an e-mail to the entire energy healing community warning them about this practitioner? Or do good ethics require that you do both? Or neither? Just what do you do?

Thinking It Through

You hear gossip by a group of practitioners about another practitioner's professional behaviors. Are you required to take action? Guidelines that might be relevant in this case include:

1. When you believe there may have been an ethical violation by another energy healing practitioner, you attempt to resolve the issue by bringing it to the attention of that individual if an informal resolution appears possible and appropriate. Such interventions may not, however, violate any confidentiality rights that are involved. *(The Resolution of Ethical Issues—1)*

2. You show respect for various personalities, rhythms, representational styles, educational levels, and backgrounds; do not falsely impugn the reputation of your colleagues; and do not file or encourage the filing of ethics complaints that are made with disregard for facts that would disprove the allegation. *(The Resolution of Ethical Issues—5)*

3. You treat colleagues with dignity, respect, and courtesy; resist gossip; and talk about colleagues in respectful ways. *(Personal and Interpersonal Boundaries—12)*

Nina McIntosh wisely observed in *The Educated Heart* (p. 80): "We all have ex-clients who think we're skilled and compassionate and those who do not. Take care with another practitioner's reputation." As you clarify your primary responsibilities in this situation, supporting the well-being and effectiveness of the colleague in question and the consequent welfare of his or her clients is primary.

But you are not in direct contact with the colleague or his or her clients. Rather, you are part of a group of practitioners that are, with whatever degree of good intent, gossiping about their colleague's treatment choices. You do not know their sources of information or whether they have discussed their concerns with the colleague. Since this kind of gossip is already violating several ethical principles, you are called upon to demonstrate "a personal commitment to acting ethically" by encouraging ethical behavior in your colleagues. You can point out that the discussion does not seem to be treating the colleague "with dignity, respect, and courtesy" and steer it toward the ethical steps those with the concerns can now take.

The first step is for them to review or verify their information and its sources and, if valid and reflecting inappropriate treatment, obtain as much permission as possible to share it with their colleague. The information they have may already ethically require them to involve themselves in the situation. Though they cannot break confidentiality, they can explain to the source of the information the importance of being able to cite a source if action is to be taken that will help correct the problem and protect other prospective clients.

The second step is for them to speak respectfully with the colleague, presenting information, but also entering with an open mind, without having formed firm conclusions. The colleague's response should be listened to with courtesy and respect. If it appears that the colleague's treatment choices are creating harm, potentially creating harm, or likely to create harm, further action is called for.

It may be possible to resolve the situation on the basis of these discussions. Those expressing the concerns need to feel confident that appropriate steps are being taken so the problems will not repeat themselves and that appropriate restitution is or will be made to the clients involved. Reaching this level of resolution might, if the practitioner in question is open to it, involve those who expressed the concerns engaging with the person in problem-solving, which might lead, for instance, to the person establishing formal consultation about the issues involved.

If resolution cannot be reached and there is substantiated concern about harm being done, the next step is to take the issue to an ethics committee. Such committees were created, in part, to weigh existing evidence when other steps have not succeeded and to intervene if necessary. It is a very serious step for a practitioner to report to an ethics committee a complaint against another practitioner; every means possible to resolve the situation should be explored prior to taking that step.

In this vignette, if the colleagues gossiping about the person refuse to take action after you lay out the ethical steps outlined here, they themselves may be engaging in unethical behavior and you are called upon to bring the discussion to focus on that possibility.

This case raises a related issue, which is the wildfire power of e-mail and blog gossip. "Groupthink" can become rampant. Aside from the studies showing that e-mails about emotional issues are more likely to be misinterpreted than to be understood in the way the sender intended, the isolation of writing an e-mail makes it easy to use words that unintentionally exaggerate your feelings or your position. The one-way nature of writing an e-mail as contrasted with a live discussion, in which you get continual visual and auditory feedback, exacerbates the problem. Emotions you might never express in person may seem safer to express in an e-mail yet do a great deal of unanticipated damage. Be very cautious about attacking anyone via e-mail, directly or indirectly. You are leaving a record that might reflect your emotion of the moment, but if presented to you a month later, or presented to others, it may evoke the common reaction of "What was I thinking?" You are wise to use the most stringent ethical language possible when engaging in electronic communication, and it may also help keep you on the best track to imagine that the person you are characterizing is sitting in front of you.

CASE VIGNETTE 28

You have an intense session with a new client, which includes substantial neurolymphatic work. The next day the client calls you. She feels terrible, is running a 102-degree temperature, believes your session is responsible for it, and wants you to come right over to her home to give her a free session to ease the aftermath of your original session. What do you do?

Thinking It Through

You have provided services consistent with your training. The client is feeling ill the next day, has concluded that your session was responsible for this, and wants you to come to her home to provide a free emergency session. Guidelines that might be relevant in this case are:

1. You hold as the highest priority the health and welfare of your client. *(General Principles—1)*

2. You open yourself to feedback offered by your clients. *(Personal Healing and Development—5)*

3. You utilize an informed consent form or other device to provide clear information to prospective clients about the nature of your services. *(Informed Consent—1)*

4. You ensure that your clients understand and agree to the specifics in the informed consent form before commencing energy healing services. *(Informed Consent—2)*

5. You engage each client in identifying goals for the services being sought and mutually create an appropriate plan of care, which may, as appropriate, include engaging other health-care professionals. *(The Healing Relationship—1)*

6. You recognize that clear, compassionate communication is integral to providing the highest level of service possible and act accordingly. *(Personal and Interpersonal Boundaries—3)*

7. You use your own professional judgment on the kinds of intake information, assessments, interventions, and session-by-session outcomes you record and maintain in the client's file. *(Record Keeping—2)*

Because your client believes you have done her harm, your actions here may have future consequences for you. Rather than assuming a defensive posture, however, a more auspicious attitude is to take this situation as an opportunity to establish a stronger healing bond between you and this new client.

Though you do not know whether the session brought about your client's symptoms, it is a possibility. The body can go into a temporary reaction after healing work that will ultimately be beneficial. But in any case, your client does not know that and is certainly not experiencing her symptoms as a potentially beneficial outcome. Begin by carefully listening to her concerns and validating her experience while also bringing your perspective to the situation. You have a line to walk here between becoming defensive about or unresponsive to the accusation that you caused the problem (along with the demand that you immediately fix it) versus becoming overly accommodating.

Your client's immediate physical state and 102-degree temperature must be taken seriously. It is not within your scope of practice to treat a high temperature, and your first advice should be geared toward ensuring that she is attending appropriately to the 102-degree temperature. Once you are assured that critical medical issues are being managed, you can explore what occurred during the session, what is occurring now, the possible connections between the two, and appropriate next steps.

You will have a better foundation for this discussion if your informed consent form addresses such "healing crises" or if you alerted your client during the session, when you realized that it was an intense session, that sometimes when considerable energy is moved during a session, the body may react.

You can discuss the woman's physical response as potentially being part of the release and integration process of energy work, while also acknowledging that it may be unrelated to the energy work. People do get the flu. Regardless of the cause of the current symptoms, which may never be decisively established, compassion is in order.

You also have several judgment calls to make here. Though your client's health and welfare are your highest priority, conveying that the session was harmful if it was not (e.g., if this is a healing crisis or an unrelated illness) does not serve your client or your future work together. Providing clear and accurate information about likely possibilities does.

If, however, you feel that you were negligent, your professional conscience must dictate the kinds of restitution you are willing to provide (e.g., free session, immediate response, house call). Though house calls are not in themselves unethical, they do create boundary issues that are easily avoided by holding even emergency sessions in your professional office. This is a new client who is already upset with you, so maintaining all reasonable professional boundaries is advisable.

Even if you do not feel you were negligent, you may want to accommodate your client's requests as much as possible. You might not provide an immediate free session at the client's home, but you might insert her into your schedule at your earliest convenience for a session in your office where you are compensated for your professional time, or you may be even more accommodating. All of the issues involved regarding when, where, and fees charged provide opportunities to establish more clearly the nature of the professional healing relationship with this new client.

In the immediate situation of the phone call, you also have tools you can offer over the phone. Specific energy techniques are indicated by her symptoms; for example, techniques are available for flushing out released toxins. These might all be explored, with verbal guidance as she carries them out, and assessment of their immediate impact on how she feels dictating next steps.

Document the entire interaction in the client's file and, if the matter was not resolved to your client's satisfaction, you would be wise to consult with a colleague and enter that discussion into your notes as well. This is a case in which the potential that the client might file a complaint against you is relatively high. The consultation would both review what occurred and explore steps you still might take toward resolving the matter.

CASE VIGNETTE 29

When doing an energy session with a male client, a female practitioner becomes aware her client has a noticeable erection. What would be an appropriate and ethical way to deal with this?

Thinking It Through

This may be an unremarkable situation or it may involve interpersonal dimensions that warrant attention. Relevant guidelines include:

1. You recognize that energy healing may open issues that are private, delicate, or embarrassing. You should be prepared to articulate these issues when they emerge and discuss them in a frank, professional, and respectful manner, while at the same time acknowledging the client's right not to discuss the issue. *(Personal and Interpersonal Boundaries—4)*

2. Dual relationships that are never acceptable are ones in which a practitioner develops any kind of romantic or sexual relationship with a client while energy healing services are being provided. *(Personal and Interpersonal Boundaries—17)*

3. You closely monitor your need to be liked, to be admired, to achieve status, and to exercise power, as well as your sexual and romantic needs, and seek feedback, guidance, consultation, and supervision from friends, colleagues, mentors, supervisors, or other professionals to keep these needs from interfering with your effectiveness in the services you provide. *(Personal Healing and Development—6)*

Because erections occur periodically with no apparent stimulus or can be caused by moving energy with no sexual dimension, no particular response is initially required on your part. If it is apparent to the client that his erection is obvious to you, or if you sense feelings of embarrassment or awkwardness in the client or in you, you might make an objective, normalizing statement, such as "When energies move through the body, it is not unusual for a man to have an erection." You also have the option of using techniques that require the man to lie face down in order to minimize his sense of embarrassment or exposure.

If the man's erections become an impediment to the sessions, or an ongoing response, sexual attraction toward you may be involved. Your choices here need to be made with great sensitivity. The man may have no intention of acting on his attraction and may truly feel it is none of your business or may be enormously embarrassed about it. Or he may be unashamedly communicating to you his attraction and his intentions. Various other cues will give you some basis to sense where he is on this spectrum, but the initial situation remains that his erections are starting to impact the sessions.

At this point, comment and inquiry are called for, speaking in honest and compassionate terms and attempting to allay any embarrassment on either his part or yours. You may want to think through this possibility in advance of it ever happening so that you are able to address it in an appropriate and professional manner and can begin to desensitize yourself to potentially embarrassing elements. Role-playing with a colleague can be a very effective way of preparing yourself.

If the erections are unwanted by the client and he has no confusion about the boundaries of a professional relationship, acknowledging the situation is usually all that is needed to diffuse it. If the client is having fantasies about you or is wishing to enter a personal/romantic relationship with you, a different level of response is required. It is not unusual for a person to develop a crush on or sexual attraction toward a caregiver. While receiving this information with understanding and compassion and perhaps acknowledging the compliment involved, the next order of business is to be crystal clear that this relationship will not evolve into a romantic or sexual relationship. This can be done kindly, compassionately, and with the shield of the professional relationship as the reason you would not even consider a personal involvement, but it must also be done clearly and decisively.

This is also a time for you to look within and explore whether you have developed sexual or romantic feelings toward the client or whether your need to be liked or desired is at play in some subtle ways. If so, and again, this is human, these personal feelings should be submitted to self-reflection or discussed with a colleague or counselor and not be allowed to infiltrate your relationship with your client.

Assuming you have dealt with any personal responses that may hinder your effectiveness in resolving the issues involved, and that the client's ongoing attraction to you is impacting the healing relationship, you would next take steps to generate, with the client, appropriate strategies for addressing the situation. While acknowledging the client's right to not discuss an issue, you also need to clarify your professional role and obligations, emphasizing that your pursuing the discussion is not to be confused for sexual interest and is not a form of sexual harassment. Having your client attain full benefit from your energy healing sessions is always the underlying purpose of the discussion.

Upon understanding that there is no possible route from the professional relationship to a sexual or romantic relationship, the client has some options. Often these external professional boundaries, unambiguously conveyed, help place boundaries on the client's internal feelings and fantasies. If the client is not able to contain the feelings and they continue to interfere with the energy healing sessions, the self-sabotage involved can sometimes be productively addressed. Rather than obtaining health benefits that are available to him, he is focusing his attention and pursuit on something that is not available.

If after doing all you can to process his feelings in a manner that best serves his health and well-being and the sessions are still hampered by his feelings or fantasies, you could, with his permission, bring a consultant to a session or you could terminate the relationship while offering an appropriate referral, making clear that his best interests are your reason for doing so. If a situation emerges in which you begin to feel afraid of your client, it is appropriate to terminate the relationship and to take whatever steps are necessary to ensure your safety.

This is another situation in which, if the relationship becomes strained, you would want to keep particularly detailed records of your discussions with the client and any consultations with colleagues or a supervisor.

CASE VIGNETTE 30

In a phone interview before a first session with a woman who is seeking help for fibromyalgia, you suspect that she may have a mental disorder or an addiction to illicit drugs. You have no special training, background, or license to treat addictions or serious psychological problems. How should you proceed?

Thinking It Through

You have learned that the person wishing to work with you has problems that are beyond your scope of practice, yet these problems could impact your work together. On the other hand, you have resources that might help this person cope better with the mental health challenges being faced. Relevant guidelines include:

1. You provide services only in those areas in which you have received education, training, supervised experience, or other study that qualifies you for providing those services. *(Competence and Scope of Practice—1)*

2. You do not diagnose or treat illness unless you are simultaneously credentialed in a health discipline that allows you to do so. *(Competence and Scope of Practice—5)*

3. You ensure that prospective clients understand and agree to the specifics in their informed consent form before commencing energy healing services. *(Informed Consent—2)*

4. You are committed to give all persons access to and benefit from the contributions of energy healing, while retaining the right to maintain your own integrity, best judgment, and personal safety at all times. *(General Principles—8)*

5. You engage each client in identifying goals for the services being sought and mutually create an appropriate plan of care, which may include engaging other health-care professionals. *(The Healing Relationship—1)*

6. You do not overstate the power of your methods. *(The Healing Relationship—4)*

7. You elicit each client's hopes and expectations for using energy healing, and discuss any unrealistic expectations as early in the healing relationship as is reasonable before providing services. Expectations are reevaluated throughout the professional relationship. *(The Healing Relationship—5)*

8. You exercise the right to refuse to accept into your care any person seeking your services when you judge this not to be in the best interests of the client. *(The Healing Relationship—7)*

9. You consult with, refer to, or cooperate with other professionals and institutions to the extent needed to serve the best interests of your clients. In particular, you understand the boundaries and limitations of your services and make referrals accordingly. *(The Healing Relationship—8)*

Signs that you are dealing with a serious psychological problem include incoherent, slurred, or rapid speech; lack of affect or persistent emotional overwhelm; disorientation; signs of delusion or paranoia; evidence of self-destructive behavior or substance abuse; or various kinds of interpersonal idiosyncrasies. You would want to learn very early of the person's previous treatment for psychiatric disorders, use of medications, use of addictive substances, and any history of suicidal or violent behavior. Since she is not asking for help with her psychological problems, however, this assessment is to determine whether such problems might interfere with your work on the energetic basis of her fibromyalgia, not whether you can treat her schizophrenia, cocaine addiction, or other psychological problem.

This early assessment not only anticipates ways that mental disorders might become an obstacle to her physical healing, but also establishes a foundation for discussing them if they do. In rare cases, you may feel you are over your head, or that working with this person might lead to unpredictable or even dangerous behavior, and you may decide not to continue to work with the person. A referral to a mental health professional or other health-care practitioner would be appropriate. A more likely possibility is that you would insist on working in conjunction with a mental health professional, with release of information forms signed and the opportunity for mutual consultation established. Because serious psychological problems may interfere with your work together, this relationship with her counselor may become a vital resource at a later point.

As always, you would begin by listening carefully to the client's expectations and goals and, together, create an appropriate plan of care. Also as always, when actually working with her, your focus is to assess where her energy systems need attention and to provide those energy systems with that care while also educating her about how to maintain the benefits with back-home follow-up.

CASE VIGNETTE 31

While at a local restaurant in your small town, you overhear two energy healing practitioners discussing a client. Even though they don't reveal a name, you recognize by the description of the problem the person they are discussing. What are you obligated to do?

Thinking It Through

You have inadvertently overheard a discussion in a public setting detailing confidential details about a client's health care. This breach of ethics came to your attention during your personal rather than professional activities and without the knowledge of the practitioners involved. Relevant guidelines include:

1. When consulting with colleagues, energy healing practitioners do not disclose confidential information that could reasonably lead to the identification of a client with whom they have a confidential relationship, unless they have obtained the prior consent of the person or the disclosure cannot be avoided. Informed consent forms may include a stipulation that the practitioner can seek supervision or consultation about the client. *(Confidentiality—3)*

2. If you believe there may have been an ethical violation by another energy healing practitioner, you attempt to resolve the issue by bringing it to the attention of that individual if an informal resolution appears possible and appropriate. If the issue is not adequately resolved through these informal steps, you take further action appropriate to the circumstances. Such action might include informing the relevant ethics committee of the situation. *(The Resolution of Ethical Issues—1, 2)*

3. You treat colleagues with dignity, respect, and courtesy. *(Personal and Interpersonal Boundaries—12)*

4. Energy healing practitioners open themselves to feedback offered by their colleagues. *(Personal Healing and Development—5)*

The practitioners have unwittingly violated professional ethics in that their conversation revealed the identity of a client, as well as information from the client's sessions, to at least one individual (you) who is not involved in the case. You also do not know if the client's practitioner had consent to be discussing this client with a colleague in a manner that could reasonably lead to knowing the client's identity, but for the purposes of this discussion, we will assume that the practitioner's informed consent form allowed such discussion with colleagues or supervisors.

The dilemma in this scenario is whether it is your responsibility to act as a policing agent for energy healing ethics. Although you have agreed to intervene or inform appropriate ethics bodies if you have knowledge of ethical violations by fellow energy healing practitioners, this situation puts all involved in an awkward position. After all, you were, however innocently, listening in on a conversation that the other two practitioners believed was being held in a quiet and confidential mode. On the other hand, even if you were listening in on what was believed to be a private conversation, others could have overheard as well, and the practitioners need to know that they were talking in a venue and at a volume and with enough details as to violate confidentiality.

Even though it might be embarrassing to admit that you overheard them, that is exactly what happened. Depending on the circumstances, you might go directly over to their table and respectfully explain what just occurred. You could also give them the benefit of the doubt, saying (assuming this is true) that you are sure they didn't intend for anyone to hear but you thought they'd want to know that their conversation could be overheard. If circumstances don't allow you to address the situation in the moment, you could later privately contact one or both of them.

In almost all cases, this will resolve the ethical dilemma. They will probably be surprised that they could be overheard, let you know that they were totally unaware of the breach, express some level of chagrin, and assure you that this will not happen again, lesson learned, thank you! If, on the other hand, you receive an angry response or a "mind your own business" reply, you have cause for concern. Is there reason to believe that rather than quietly conducting a consultation, they were gossiping about the client in a cavalier manner, inattentive to confidentiality issues, not caring who heard what was said? If after your conversation, you feel they were being callous about the confidentiality issue, this suddenly escalates from an innocent case of carelessness to a serious disregard of ethical principles. In that case, you may state your dilemma that as a certified energy healing practitioner, you are duty-bound to get a better resolution than has so far occurred, with taking the situation to the appropriate ethics committee being a last resort.

CASE VIGNETTE 32

After meeting with a client several times, you are asked to attend a Worker's Compensation hearing regarding a disability the client is claiming. Even though your case notes from a few months earlier did not

comment on various issues relevant to the hearing, you feel confident that you can reconstruct your notes, adding pertinent details for the benefit of the hearing. Should you do this?

Thinking It Through

You did not anticipate that you would need to present formal case notes on this client, but you are apparently now being called upon to produce them. You remember the sessions well enough that you feel you could accurately introduce pertinent details retrospectively. Should you? Relevant guidelines include:

1. Regarding whether to reconstruct your notes, the guidelines are clear: "Do not alter records. Additions that correct earlier information should be dated." *(Record Keeping—4)*

2. When energy healing practitioners are required by law, institutional policy, or extraordinary circumstances to serve in more than one role in judicial or administrative proceedings, they clarify role expectations and the extent of confidentiality as early as possible. *(Personal and Interpersonal Boundaries—16)*

3. Your client (or the client's legal guardian or conservator) is the only person who has the right to determine who has access to information about the energy healing services he or she has received from you, including the very question of whether a person is receiving such services from you. *(Confidentiality—1)*

You are prohibited from altering your notes. You can, however, introduce additions or corrections with the date of the entry clearly noted. You must also carefully monitor your impartiality. Despite the potential temptation to do so, you cannot ethically add comments just to help your client get a desired ruling.

The request to attend the hearing brings up a number of other issues about the interface between your energy healing practice setting and the outside community. Are you legally required to attend the hearing? If it is not a legal requirement, what are your client's wishes? If it is a requirement that you attend, does your client give you written permission to disclose your observations? If not, be sure you understand how local law impacts privileged information for your type of practice. If you are required to attend the hearing, are you required to attend it on your own time or can you bill the client or the government agency for your time? Such considerations can be thought through in advance of establishing a practice, perhaps with legal consultation, and can be included in your informed consent form.

If attending the hearing is not a legal requirement, and you feel that your testimony will hurt your client's chances for the desired settlement, you might take extra measures to emphasize strongly that while you will always do your best to be supportive of your client, you are ethically bound to be honest and to maintain your professional observations rather than to take an advocacy position. You should also emphasize that it is your client's choice whether to involve you, but if you do become involved, you cannot guarantee any outcome. You might also consider discussing how the client would feel if you did present information and the claim was denied and how that might impact future energy healing sessions with you.

CASE VIGNETTE 33

After seeing a client for more than a year, you feel satisfied with her progress and feel you have little more to offer. When you talk to the client about ending your work together, she becomes very upset and you learn that she has a strong emotional attachment to you and wants to continue to work with you. What do you do?

Thinking It Through

You have helped this woman as much as you feel you can in achieving the health goals for which she has been coming to you. She wants to continue to work with you because of the strong emotional attachment she has developed for you. Relevant guidelines include:

1. You may attempt to encourage, but you do not attempt to pressure or coerce a client into any action or belief. *(The Healing Relationship—3)*

2. You elicit each client's hopes and expectations for using energy healing. You also discuss any unrealistic expectations as early in the healing relationship as is reasonable. *(The Healing Relationship—5)*

3. You consult with, refer to, or cooperate with other professionals to the extent needed to serve the best interests of your clients. *(The Healing Relationship—8)*

4. You may terminate a client relationship when it becomes reasonably clear that the client no longer needs or is no longer benefiting from the continued service. *(The Healing Relationship—18)*

5. You closely monitor your needs to be liked and admired, and seek feedback and consultation from friends, colleagues, or other professionals to keep those needs from interfering with your effectiveness in the services you provide. *(Personal Healing and Development—6)*

6. You engage each client in identifying goals for the services being sought and mutually create an appropriate plan of care. *(The Healing Relationship—1)*

Deep emotional attachments to a healer or other nurturing figure are not unusual, nor are they necessarily undesirable. They are often part of the road to physical and emotional self-empowerment. You should nonetheless be alert for this dynamic, articulate it in a respectful way that makes it a theme for reflection while still acknowledging the value of trusting and accepting guidance from a healer, and that also encourages and instructs people toward achieving increasing independence.

In this case, the attachment developed beneath your radar. You would begin by very sensitively exploring the client's feelings about you and expectations regarding a continuing relationship. Is this friendship-for-pay by someone who is extremely lonely; is it lack of confidence in being able to maintain the healing gains that have been achieved; is it a sexual attraction? What hopes or fantasies are involved? Your next step depends on the nature of the client's emotional attachment to you, but in none of these circumstances would you end the relationship abruptly.

If it is a situation in which you are the only friend in the life of an isolated person, you would, with the client, map out steps for addressing the person's social needs in more appropriate ways. As this moves into the realm of psychotherapy, you must be very careful if you are not a psychotherapist to stay within your scope of practice. Referral to a psychotherapist would definitely be an option to consider. But you still have a number of ways to proceed that do not move into "treating" a "mental disorder." You have been working with this woman for a year, and a review of how your relationship with her has developed could lead to insights that are important to her and reveal viable next steps in her development. If you have training in energy psychology, you can teach her how to apply it to address her fear of meeting people, to reduce her anxiety about the thought of not continuing to work with you, and to strengthen the impact of affirmations regarding taking other steps to meet her interpersonal needs.

If it is a situation in which she is afraid that she will not be able to maintain the healing gains if she is not seeing you, this is a totally different kind of dependence. Because it is less emotionally charged, the solutions can be more straightforward. You could, for instance, put much more emphasis on her back-home assignments and educate her on how to assess their impact and how to formulate new routines as appropriate. You could gradually reduce the frequency of sessions. You could suggest written material or video resources. You could encourage her to join a study group or take classes. All of these will bolster realistic confidence and independence through tried experience.

If her emotional dependence is a matter of sexual attraction or romantic fantasies, while exploring the client's feelings with compassion and respect, you must also be crystal clear in communicating that there is no chance of this becoming a sexual or romantic relationship. Some of the issues are similar to those in the second half of the discussion of vignette 29, such as examining your own feelings that may be confusing the situation and processing them outside of your relationship with the client. Once having set unambiguous boundaries and having become clear about your own motivations, you can begin, with the client, to map out steps for handling the situation that she is attracted to someone who is not available and is not reciprocating. Romance does not stay as compelling when examined under a microscope, and if the client is willing, a frank discussion of the progression of her feelings and fantasies in the context of what else is going on in her life can be extremely useful in moving her beyond what is for her a dead end. Referring her for counseling could lead to the same benefits, though making the referral might be interpreted as dumping or abandoning her. In some cases, when a client becomes extremely distraught or aggressive, it may be valuable to bring a consultant into a session to help map a strategy for bringing the relationship to as constructive a conclusion as possible. Throughout all this, keep an open, sensitive, and respectful dialogue going with the client.

CASE VIGNETTE 34

You have a session with a client who has just left an abusive husband and is living in a safe house. Her fears, memories, and physiological reactions quickly surface and become a central part of your work together. You find that you are strongly triggered by feelings from some old personal history around similar issues. What do you do?

Thinking It Through

It is not unusual for a client's emotional wounds to touch us deeply and, sometimes, personal issues that are unresolved or unhealed will be triggered in ways that could potentially interfere with our services. Called "countertransference" in psychotherapy, this phenomenon can impact any form of intimate healing work. Since we are human first and practitioners second, with our own histories of trauma and vulnerabilities, instances of countertransference are likely to affect us at various times in our careers. When they do, relevant guidelines include:

1. You hold as the highest priority the health and welfare of your client. *(General Principles—1)*

2. You know your limitations as an individual and as a practitioner. *(Personal Healing and Development—4)*

3. You monitor the effects of your own physical health, mental state, and ego needs on your ability to help those with whom you work and take appropriate steps to maximize your well-being in each area. *(Personal Healing and Development—2)*

4. You consult with, refer to, or cooperate with other professionals and institutions to the extent needed to serve the best interests of your clients. *(The Healing Relationship—8)*

The obvious first step is to make a personal assessment of the ways your responses to your client's issues are impacting you and the healing relationship. This may be as simple as making a mental or written note during the session about what triggered you and taking time after the session to work mindfully with it or journal about it until you have resolved the issue for yourself prior to the next session.

Sometimes, however, you are not readily able to resolve a counter-transference issue through mindfulness or inner reflection. At that point, you may want to discuss your reactions with a trusted colleague or a counselor. Subjecting your feelings to discussion adds a level of objectivity to the way you respond to them. With your client's health and welfare as your highest priority, you have several decisions to make:

1. Are you capable of continuing to work with the client without your own reactions hindering the quality of services you are able to provide?
2. Do you need extra support, such as psychotherapy or formal supervision, to deal with the feelings that have been triggered in you?
3. If you do continue to work with the client without engaging in psychotherapy or formal supervision, how will you continue to monitor the situation? You might, for instance, arrange for ongoing reality checks with the colleague you first consulted.

The question of whether to share your countertransference or personal history with your client is also likely to occur to you. This can be delicate. The energy healing sessions are for your client's healing, not yours. Though your healing is certainly important, your client's sessions are not the setting for the vast majority of that process. In fact, you should generally refrain from disclosing your own issues if they are relatively raw. Once you do have some traction in your own healing process, sharing analogous stories from your own life may acknowledge an energetic or emotional aspect of your relationship with the client that has been occurring without acknowledgment. It can also be a way of communicating empathy around one of the client's core traumas. Sharing can be normalizing and affirming, and to the degree that you have healed regarding the issue, it can be inspiring. Discussion with a colleague, supervisor, or therapist on how much to disclose, if anything, would be called for in the situation presented in this case vignette.

You may decide you are too raw regarding your own vulnerabilities to address your client's issues effectively. In this case, strong sensitivity and diplomacy are called for. The woman has shared one of her deepest wounds with you and may now feel punished or rejected for having done so. You need to provide enough information so she is not likely to come to these kinds of erroneous conclusions while at the same time not making yourself a cause for the woman's sympathy or guilt. Discussing in advance, or even rehearsing how you will do this with a consultant, as well as identifying the most suitable referral sources, can help ensure that this delicate process is done appropriately and well.

CASE VIGNETTE 35

You feel good about your client's progress and the work you are doing together. The client expresses feeling great compassion and caring coming from you. A few sessions later, the client admits to feeling a strong romantic attraction toward you. You explain a bit about transference, but later you find that the discussion has sparked your own romantic interest. You are both single and available. Can you become friendlier and continue to work together? Should you refer the client to another practitioner so that you can pursue a personal relationship? Is there any reason you should not explore an opportunity for a meaningful relationship?

Thinking It Through

Not only has your client developed romantic feelings toward you, but you also find your own heart reciprocating. The intimacy of your work together has been intense, you have come to know this person at a soul level, and you are drawn toward exploring whether your life partner has appeared to you in the somewhat inconvenient context of your energy healing practice. You vaguely remember that there are professional guidelines for this kind of situation and reluctantly review them. You find that:

1. Dual relationships that are never acceptable are ones in which a practitioner develops any kind of romantic or sexual relationship with a client while energy healing services are being provided. *(Personal and Interpersonal Boundaries—17)*

2. You do not engage in sexual relations with a former client for at least a year after termination of the client relationship, and only then after a good faith determination through appropriate consultation that there is no exploitation of the former client. *(Personal and Interpersonal Boundaries—18)*

3. You closely monitor your needs to be liked, to be admired, to achieve status, and to exercise power, as well as your sexual and romantic needs, and seek feedback, guidance, consultation, and supervision from friends, colleagues, mentors, supervisors, or other professionals to keep these needs from interfering with your effectiveness in the services you provide. *(Personal Healing and Development—6)*

4. If you find that, due to unforeseen factors, a potentially harmful dual relationship has arisen, you take reasonable steps to resolve it with due regard for the best interests of the affected person and maximal compliance with the "Ethics Code for Energy Healing Practitioners." *(Personal and Interpersonal Boundaries—15)*

5. Energy healing practitioners who reach an interpersonal impasse with a client, or an impasse in the healing services they are providing, may seek supervision, suggest bringing a consultant into a session, refer the client to another practitioner, or suggest terminating their services. *(The Healing Relationship—19)*

Seeing nothing in the previous that would ethically prevent you from pursuing your romantic interests, you are reminded that "the mind, even of a sincere professional health-care provider, can powerfully rationalize inappropriate behavior when driven by romantic and/or sexual desire" (from vignette 8).

The entire discussion in vignette 8, in fact, applies here as well. As noted there: "At a minimum, when romantic/sexual feelings or fantasies about a client persist, your first step should be to inform a colleague and enter a formal or informal supervisory relationship with your colleague about this case.... Often, bringing in a consultant or supervisor will itself shift the energy for you. The power of being unambiguously watched by the entire profession, through the concerned eyes of one of its members, has a way of cooling ardor, as does the commitment it represents of placing professional ethics above personal impulse. Self-examination of the needs and/or unresolved emotional issues this client is triggering in you may also be personally illuminating."

The guidelines themselves are unambiguous. You have no ethical leeway to "become friendlier" or "explore an opportunity for a meaningful relationship." Your practice is never to be allowed to become a source for meeting your romantic needs. Your primal desires cannot be given more credence than the collective experience of generations of health-care providers, which concludes that when a practitioner crosses sexual or romantic boundaries, the healing relationship is compromised, the client is frequently harmed, and the sanctity of the healing setting as a safe haven is diminished. Respecting such boundaries was a commitment you made when you accepted the public trust of opening an energy healing practice.

While all the principles from vignette 8 apply here, the primary difference is that in this situation the client is having and has disclosed romantic feelings toward you. You may feel a desire to indicate that those feelings are not unrequited, to signal that your client is not alone in something beautiful that is developing between the two of you. And after all, aren't you ethically bound to offer honest disclosure?

In this case, the more fundamental principle, and more so now than ever, is to maintain a firm boundary with the client regarding any romantic involvement. The client absolutely needs this to manage appropriately the feelings and fantasies that are arising about you. Sharing your own feelings in this situation starts to cross and blur the romantic boundaries, implicitly encouraging and even enticing the client toward a relationship that is not possible.

Though it is not appropriate in this case to disclose your feelings to your client, it is highly appropriate and strongly recommended that you discuss them with a close friend, trusted colleague, supervisor, or therapist. As discussed in vignette 33, "Romance does not stay as compelling when examined under a microscope." You have some serious self-examination ahead of you. Questions posed in vignette 8 that are also relevant here include: "What is occurring within you that is straining the limits of your professional commitments and threatening your entire professional life? What unmet personal needs are spilling into your professional relationships? How can you better meet them? What unresolved emotional issue is this client tapping into?" You might also be curious about the timing of your romantic interest, emerging only after the client's was revealed. Asking these kinds of questions can—often with the aid of a psychotherapist, supervisor, colleague, or close friend—ultimately serve your personal evolution.

Once you begin to understand your feelings, you may be able to "bracket" them (keep them out of your sessions with the client). This makes it possible for you to continue the healing relationship. In terms of your commitment to the client's health and welfare, this would be a desirable course of action since the two of you were making good progress in the healing work and it would allow an opportunity for the client's emotional response to you to be fully processed for the client's benefit. In some cases, your feelings may remain intense and not go through a healthy transmutation after examination. They may be interfering with the healing relationship. Conversely, you may succeed in bracketing your feelings, but the client may pursue you romantically and refuse to take no for an answer. In such instances, you might, with the client's concurrence, bring a consultant into one of the sessions to assess the situation and provide recommendations for next steps. Where you have been successful in bracketing your feelings, but your client has not, you might need to refer the client to a psychotherapist instead of, or as a condition of, continuing to work with you.

If you find through your self-examination or counseling that you are unable to contain your attraction toward the client, you are obligated to end the professional relationship. You cannot, however, do this for the purpose of then entering a romantic relationship. The "One-Year Rule" *(Personal and Interpersonal Boundaries—18)* is designed to ensure that terminating a professional relationship is not simply a ploy to move into a romantic or sexual one.

However, to continue to see the client when you cannot contain your attraction violates your commitment to take effective action when your own mental state interferes with the services you are providing. If consultation or therapy has not helped you resolve your part of the interpersonal impasse, you are obligated to suggest terminating the services. Referral to another practitioner would be appropriate. The way you explain your reasoning is delicate. Your reasoning has to do with the romantic feelings that have entered the office and your discomfort or inability to work with them constructively. You are in a bind. You cannot express your own romantic feelings (as this may encourage your client's romantic interest), nor may you imply that it is the client's fault that a referral to another practitioner is needed. The wording you find for this unique situation is important and may grow out of a consultative relationship in which you have a chance to brainstorm, rehearse, and receive feedback.

This is another case where you would be well advised to keep particularly detailed records of the conversations you have with the client regarding the situation, as well as with any colleagues or supervisors you involve. The way the client responds to your explanation of why you are making a referral might not be predictable. The client may, for instance, feel rejected by you and may make untrue accusations about your conduct. Having records and someone else aware of the situation will be useful should you have to defend your conduct.

CASE VIGNETTE 36

You are deeply involved in working with a woman with multiple sclerosis and her physician is impressed with the results. The woman's brother has been driving her to the sessions and you have been enjoying brief chats before and after the sessions. The brother invites you to lunch, with clear romantic overtones. You are both unpartnered, and you are interested. Can you pursue this relationship? If your attraction is very strong, but you decide you cannot simultaneously work with the woman and pursue the relationship, can you refer the woman to another practitioner?

Thinking It Through

This vignette differs from the previous one in that your attraction is toward a relative of your client rather than your client. Does this give you leeway to explore the relationship? Relevant guidelines include:

1. You hold as the highest priority in your professional activities the health and welfare of your client. *(General Principles—1)*

2. You do not enter into a dual relationship that could reasonably be expected to impair your objectivity, competence, or effectiveness in the delivery of healing or educational services. *(Personal and Interpersonal Boundaries—13)*

3. Dual relationships that would not reasonably be expected to cause impairment or risk exploitation or harm are not unethical. However, it is your responsibility to ensure that each party is aware of issues related to shifting between the client-practitioner setting and the social setting of the personal relationship. These issues should be discussed with the client and take precedence in decisions about the dual relationship. *(Personal and Interpersonal Boundaries—14)*

4. You examine your need to be liked, to be admired, to achieve status, and to exercise power, as well as your sexual and romantic needs, and seek feedback, guidance, and consultation. *(Personal Healing and Development—6)*

Your priority is your client's health and well-being. Entering a personal relationship with her brother, who is also a caregiver at least to the extent that he drives her to her sessions, is fraught with hazards. First, it signals to your client that her well-being is not your highest priority, and it backs this message with actions that could jeopardize your work with her. If things with the brother go well and the relationship blossoms into the passion of new love, your bond with the brother may become stronger than your bond with your client so she is energetically relegated to a third-wheel position each time he brings her for a session. If things with the brother start nicely and then blow up, the shrapnel will almost inevitably find its way into your relationship with your client. The rule of thumb is that you do not use your professional practice as a source for meeting your romantic needs.

So your obligation is to articulate and set a strong energetic as well as physical boundary with the brother, for the purpose of respecting the integrity of your work with your client. This may be shared with the client and, in fact, is relevant for her to know. If you are unable to take these steps without equivocation or sending a double message, a consultation or personal counseling may be called for.

Where there may be some leeway is in the fact that the "One-Year Rule" *(Personal and Interpersonal Boundaries—18)* does not apply to a family member who was never your client. Exploring a personal relationship with the brother *following the completion of your work with his sister* is not expressly prohibited. You still, however, would need to consider your former client's welfare. For instance, what if she had a setback and wanted to reengage your services? What if she felt in some way betrayed by your subsequently entering a relationship with her brother? There is also the consideration that your entering a personal relationship with her brother would almost certainly mean that you are simultaneously entering a personal relationship with your former client.

In coming to a decision when ethical regulations do not provide clear direction, the context may provide further guidance, including factors such as:

- Was your relationship with the client characterized by dependency or was there more of a sense of equality? If the former, how will that play into your becoming involved in her family?
- Has the client successfully transferred her clinical relationship to someone else, does she otherwise have adequate supports to replace

the work she did with you, or might she still need to rely on you for help with her healing?

- Will it be countertherapeutic for your former client to get to know you, "warts and all"?

- Does the client have a happy and secure partner relationship of her own?

- Does the client's multiple sclerosis appear to have a connection to her family dynamics?

- What is the nature of the relationship between the brother and your former client?

- How does your client respond when you consult her about her feelings regarding your having a personal relationship with her brother?

- Has the brother gained his sister's wholehearted agreement about dating you?

It is generally wise to maintain as strong a boundary between your professional practice and your personal life as possible, but the previous factors may all be taken into consideration in coming to a responsible decision.

CASE VIGNETTE 37

Your client reveals after your third session together that he was a victim of ritual abuse that is still a source of trauma and anxiety for him. In the next session, he has an overwhelming flashback and dissociates. You manage to help stabilize him, but the issues are clearly not resolved. You learn that he has never had therapy for these experiences, but when you recommend therapy, he claims that the cost of both entering psychotherapy and continuing to see you would be prohibitive. You have been helping him with symptoms of hypertension and overall well-being. What do you do?

Thinking It Through

You are faced with a situation in which you suspect an untreated psychological trauma is contributing to your client's current physical problems but you do not have the skills or training to provide the psychotherapy you believe is necessary. Relevant guidelines include:

1. You respect the inherent dignity, worth, and uniqueness of your clients and their right to self-determination. *(General Principles—7)*

2. You engage clients in mutually creating an appropriate plan of care, which may include engaging other health-care professionals. *(The Healing Relationship—1)*

3. You do not diagnose or treat illness unless you are simultaneously credentialed in a health discipline that allows you to do so. *(Competence and Scope of Practice—5)*

4. You provide healing, teaching, supervision, consultation, and mentoring services only in areas in which you have received education, training, supervised experience, or other study that qualifies you for providing those services. It is your responsibility to draw those lines professionally and appropriately. *(Competence and Scope of Practice—1)*

5. You may attempt to encourage, but you do not attempt to pressure or coerce a client into any action or belief, even if you believe such act or belief would serve the best interests of the client. *(The Healing Relationship—3)*

6. Though it is appropriate to encourage hope and convey confidence in energy healing methods, you do so without overstating the power of the methods. *(The Healing Relationship—4)*

7. You consult with, refer to, or cooperate with other professionals and institutions to the extent needed to serve the best interests of your clients. *(The Healing Relationship—8)*

8. You take steps to ensure that your personal biases, the boundaries of your competence, and the limitations of your expertise do not negatively impact the services you provide to your clients. *(Personal and Interpersonal Boundaries—1)*

Your energy healing sessions have triggered unresolved memories of extraordinary trauma that are beyond your training or scope of practice to treat. Your client has told you that it is financially not feasible to continue to work with you and simultaneously enter psychotherapy. If you continue to provide energy healing sessions for hypertension, the probability of triggering further flashbacks and dissociation is strong, and the possibility of them escalating makes it questionable whether it is in the client's best interests for you to continue the energy healing sessions except within the context of psychotherapy with a trauma specialist capable of working with ritual abuse.

While it is his choice whether to seek such treatment, you have the right and the responsibility not to offer further energy healing sessions if you believe they may ultimately be harmful to him. Your next step would involve crystal-clear communication. You are not rejecting him. You are not blaming him for being unable to utilize your services. You are directing him to the services that, in your professional judgment, will be the most beneficial to him.

It is entirely appropriate to take some time to explain the nature of psychotherapy and how it might impact his presenting problem to you, his hypertension. You can also review how the energy work is or is not improving the energy systems that are involved in his hypertension and how continued energy healing sessions after or in conjunction with his therapy might affect the affected energy systems.

CASE VIGNETTE 38

You attend a monthly meeting of local holistic health-care providers. You become aware that one of the members has recently added the credential of "MD" to his business card and advertising. When you inquire about the medical degree, he explains that he earned this credential from an East Indian university that offers an online medical degree, the only requirement of which is to write a twenty-five-page paper on the history of miraculous healing. A month later, you have a client who discusses her need for a new MD, says she heard about the member of your group, and asks you for a referral or an opinion. She wants a medical doctor who has a holistic orientation. What is your responsibility if any to your client, to the practitioner, to the group, and to the community?

Thinking It Through

Your client is under the impression that the health-care provider is a licensed MD. You know that despite his online credential, he is neither a licensed physician nor a medical doctor. Although you were surprised and concerned when he shamelessly told you about how he obtained his degree, you have not discussed your concerns with him. And since he does indeed have a degree that says he is an MD, you are not sure if there is a legal restriction on putting those letters after his name as long as he does not officially "diagnose" or "treat" illness. After all, many doctors who do research or administration never treat a patient, yet they can still represent themselves as MDs.

In any case, you were hoping not to involve yourself in the situation, wishfully thinking that a colleague who knew him better would, upon seeing the blatant misrepresentation, force him to deal with it. But now the situation has found its way into your office. You are not sure if it is your place to tell your client that you feel your colleague is misrepresenting himself. Relevant guidelines include:

1. You hold as the highest priority the health and welfare of your client. *(General Principles—1)*

2. You uphold professional standards of conduct and accept appropriate responsibility for your own behavior. *(General Principles—3)*

3. You demonstrate a personal commitment to acting ethically and encourage ethical behavior by students, supervisees, employees, and colleagues. *(General Principles—11)*

4. You provide services only in areas in which you have received education, training, supervised experience, or other study that qualifies you for providing those services. It is the responsibility of the practitioner to draw lines professionally. *(Competence and Scope of Practice—1)*

5. You engage your clients in mutually creating an appropriate plan of care, which may include engaging other health-care professionals. *(The Healing Relationship—1)*

6. You consult with, refer to, or cooperate with other professionals and institutions to the extent needed to serve the best interests of your clients. You are clear with clients about whether or not you have personal knowledge of the skills of a particular practitioner and encourage clients to interview prospective practitioners before committing themselves to the practitioner's care. *(The Healing Relationship—8)*

7. Energy healing practitioners do not make false, deceptive, or fraudulent statements concerning: (1) their training, experience, or competence; (2) their academic degrees; or (3) their credentials. *(Public Statements and Advertising—4)*

When your client asks about the practitioner, you have an immediate "aha" moment about why it is a good idea to intervene when you encounter an ethical violation. But you did not. Still, you have information that is directly and immediately relevant to your client's health-care decision. You could ethically state facts that are not disputed, or ask her to inquire about them, saying something like, "I understand that his medical degree is from an unaccredited foreign institution and that he is not licensed as an MD. You might first ask him about that." If she says something like, "Oh, I don't mind. I think many doctors trained in foreign universities are more open-minded than American doctors," your obligation for truthful communication would compel you to reveal that your understanding is that he was not trained in a foreign university either, but that he went through a brief online program to get his MD.

Having dealt with the situation at hand, there is still the question of whether you are obligated to act on your knowledge that he is misrepresenting his training and competence. First, you would want to find out if it is legal in your state for someone with an MD degree to use it as a credential on a business card or in advertising, whether or not the person is licensed or the degree-granting institution is accredited. Even if it is legal, an ethical dilemma exists in that the way the advertising is stated led your client to believe the man's credentials were those of a qualified medical doctor.

You are trained to attempt first to resolve ethical dilemmas with the professionals involved. You already know the man from your holistic health provider group. You could initiate a phone or in-person conversation with him that explored the situation. Even if he is not actually breaking the letter of the law in your state, you might inquire about whether he believes his training is equivalent to what the credential he is listing implies. If he is defensive or cavalier about it, you might tell him about your client's misinterpretation of his advertising and ask him how he would defend himself against a charge of "practicing medicine without a license." You might also ask him how he would feel about unwittingly putting a loved one into the care of someone with a bogus degree if the loved one had a serious health problem. If he insists that his training is adequate and that he genuinely feels no fraud is involved, but you feel differently, this would be a good time to clarify that with him. You are providing him with due warning to let him know that while he may not feel uncomfortable making these claims, you do.

If the outcome of this conversation is such that it is clear he intends to continue to misrepresent his training and competence, you are obligated as a member of the professional healing community to take the information you have another step. You would need to determine just what that step is. Since he is not an energy healing practitioner, your own ethics committee has no jurisdiction, though you could consult with it about your ethical obligations in the matter. If he is practicing under any recognized license, alerting the board that grants that license would be an appropriate step. But even if he has worded his business card and other formal statements about his services so that he is able to conduct his healing practice legally without a specific license, an ethical issue is still involved. You could register a complaint with the medical board or you could bring the issue up for discussion by the holistic health provider group of which you are both a part. This might induce the group to examine its policies around the credentials and representations of its members and the implications of these policies for the public's trust in holistic healing practitioners. That discussion might lead to a resolution of the situation since the man is part of the group, and in any case, responsibility for the next step would now be shared with other colleagues.

CASE VIGNETTE 39

A seventeen-year-old male has contacted you as a result of an article about energy healing mentioning your services, which he saw in a local alternative health newsletter. After making a preliminary appointment, he arrives with his mother. The mother, who will be paying for the session, insists on being present during the session. The young man is clearly giving signs he does not wish that arrangement. What do you do?

Thinking It Through

Your client is a minor whose apparent desire for privacy conflicts with his mother's desire to witness the session. Relevant guidelines include:

1. If you work with children or with more than one member of the same family (including "significant others"), you establish with the relevant parties at the outset (or when new family members begin to receive services from you) the kinds of information that may be shared, and with whom, and the kinds of information that may not be shared. *(Confidentiality—2)*

2. Your client (or the client's legal guardian or conservator) is the only person who has the right to determine who has access to information about the energy healing services he or she has received from you. *(Confidentiality—1)*

First of all, after reading this vignette, you will hopefully take steps so that you are never in this situation. It is a dilemma that could have been avoided. This young man is, in the eyes of the law, a minor child. During the initial phone call, from cues that indicated you were speaking with a young man, you should have verified his age and established the boundaries of confidentiality with him, keeping in mind your local laws relating to minors.

During that initial phone call, you would also likely have asked him the nature of the problem he wants help with. The next logical question would be: "Have you discussed this with either of your parents? Are they aware that you are calling me?"

What should have followed during the phone call was a frank discussion of all that is relevant of the following: (1) your possible liability in seeing him against his parents' wishes (if that is at issue); (2) the probability that his parents would want to know that there is a problem (if he did not tell his parents he was contacting you); (3) that, being nearly an adult, he could make a good case for engaging his parents' help in paying for the session while asking for confidentiality about the actual session if that is his preference; (4) that, if he is physically fearful of one or both of his parents, there are public agencies that can intervene on his behalf; (5) the possibility of you, the practitioner, having an initial discussion with one or both of his parents; and (6) the possibility of having an initial session with his mother and/or father present so that they can ask questions and allay any fears they might have, and then requesting that they not attend the next session. The question of this young man's privacy and his parents' involvement should be settled before he arrives for his first appointment.

The situation raises several auxiliary issues. Some practitioners generally do not allow a second person to sit in on a session (unless they are specifically doing couples work) because this changes the dynamics and the energy in the room. Simply having another person present brings in another energy field, the other person's agenda for the session, and the dynamic of having an audience. Even if the client says it is okay, you as the practitioner can state your own preference as well. In situations where there is an aspect of the session that might be relevant for involving the other person, such as if that person is a caregiver who should be shown the homework you are assigning, the person can be made comfortable in another room and asked in at the appropriate time.

More common than this vignette are situations in which one of the parents calls to schedule an appointment for a child or teenager. Here you can discuss up front your policies regarding the parent sitting in on the session and whether you require that the parent sign a waiver that allows you to keep what the child reveals confidential, even from the parents.

Another auxiliary issue regards confidentiality expectations if the session is a gift from one adult to another (some practitioners actually offer gift certificates). There is nothing in this situation that should compromise the client's confidentiality rights. Even a question from the giver about whether the client came for the gifted session is the client's to answer, not yours.

Case Vignette 40

A landscaper calls for an initial appointment. He has been off the job for the past three months due to an injury that is to be a focus of your work together. Once you tell him your fee, he says that he simply does not have the money but he really wants to work with you. He asks if he can do a work exchange of landscaping in repayment for sessions. You have just moved to a new home that needs landscaping. What do you say? Or what if the injured person is a single parent working for low pay at a nursing home, has no savings or health insurance, and can't possibly pay any appreciable fee, but the person can't function adequately without help for the injury?

Thinking It Through

You have the ability to provide services he needs; he has the ability to provide services you need. He wants to do this as a barter. Would such an arrangement compromise the quality of the health-care services you would deliver? Relevant guidelines include:

1. You may choose to barter for services only if this arrangement will not interfere with the quality of the services being provided and if the resulting arrangement is not exploitative to either party. *(The Healing Relationship—16)*

2. If limitations to services can be anticipated because of financial hardship, the related issues are discussed with the recipient of services as early as is feasible. You do not maintain a client relationship solely for financial reasons, but you may terminate a relationship if the client is unable or unwilling to pay for such services. Prior to any termination of services, the issues involved and possible alternatives are discussed, with the client's well-being as the highest priority. *(The Healing Relationship—14)*

3. Dual relationships that would not reasonably be expected to cause impairment or risk exploitation or harm are not unethical. However, it is the practitioner's responsibility to ensure that each party is aware of issues related to shifting from the client-practitioner setting. These issues should be discussed with the client and take precedence in decisions about the dual relationship. *(Personal and Interpersonal Boundaries—14)*

4. You ensure that prospective clients understand and agree to the specifics in their informed consent before commencing energy healing services. *(Informed Consent—2)*

5. You strive to keep your commitments and to avoid unwise, unrealistic, or unclear commitments. *(General Principles—5)*

6. You are committed to giving all persons access to and benefit from the contributions of energy healing. *(General Principles—8)*

7. You know your limitations as an individual and as a practitioner, setting your boundaries accordingly with those you serve. *(Personal Healing and Development—4)*

8. You exercise the right to refuse to accept into your care any person seeking your services when you judge this not to be in the best interests of the client. *(The Healing Relationship—7)*

9. If conflicts occur regarding your ethical obligations (such as when a client's inability to pay for services comes into conflict with your commitment to the client's welfare), you attempt to resolve these conflicts in a responsible fashion that avoids or minimizes harm, seeking consultation as appropriate. *(The Healing Relationship—15)*

Although bartering is not considered unethical, certain criteria must be met, with the fundamental concern being whether the arrangement might compromise the healing services the person receives.

So you must ask yourself if it is truly possible for both you and the client to "bracket" the two relationships. What if one of your recommendations in your healing role has to be that he refrain from the kinds of physical activities needed in the barter? Furthermore, how might it impact your attitude in the sessions if you are unhappy with his work in your garden? How might it impact his work in your garden if he is unhappy with your sessions? What if he reinjures himself while working in your garden because the arrangement caused him to commence working before he was physically ready to do so? Various subtle manipulations are invited when such a dual relationship is established. Ultimately, however, this is a judgment call. If unsure, you might consult with a colleague before finalizing your decision.

A way to make the dual relationship less problematic is to work with him first and have him provide his landscaping services after his sessions with you have been completed. Like any delayed payment arrangement, however, this puts you at risk of not being paid after a sizable debt has accumulated. It also makes it more likely for your payment to be dependent on his satisfaction with your services, an additional dynamic affecting your work with him that does not serve him or you. And it assumes his injuries are not permanent and that he will be able to resume work as a landscaper. But making the dual relationship sequential instead of simultaneous does remove many of the other potentially problematic factors inherent in dual relationships.

In exploring the arrangement you are about to establish, you might inquire about whether it is possible for him to find a paying client who needs the kinds of services he is offering to you so there is a clean monetary exchange on both sides. If this is not possible or he declines to consider it, and your determination is that the dual relationship would compromise your services to him, you are obligated to refuse to enter into the barter. You are then back to the same situation you are in when any person who does not have means to pay requests your services, such as the single-parent nursing-home caregiver mentioned in the vignette.

This is one of the more heart-wrenching sorts of dilemma you will face in your career as an energy healer. All professionals are encouraged to do some pro bono work, and you might choose this person as a recipient of free sessions or largely reduced fees. But the amount of pro bono or low-fee work that it is possible to offer is always limited by practical constraints, so it is possible you will need to tell the person up front that you require a specified fee in order to enter a professional relationship. For that eventuality, it is important to have an idea of other practitioners and services that are available in your community, including less experienced or less established practitioners who are competent or working with competent supervision, as they may be more flexible in their fees.

In looking for ways to serve those who do not have the ability to pay, other approaches that have been used by energy healing practitioners include offering the person a free or price-reduced spot in a class or study group, time-limited free services (such as six free sessions), or devoting an afternoon each week to a drop-in clinic where the only payment involves a donation box.

Additional Considerations. Informed consent standards obligate practitioners to inform new clients about their fees and to discuss the suggested frequency and likely duration of the services being requested. This should also address the expected payment if a session goes over the time allotted. When I (Donna Eden) had my practice, the sessions always ran at least ninety minutes, and I have often puzzled about how my students can be satisfied that they had the time to let the energies lead them when working within a shorter time frame, though my students' clients do still report great results from shorter sessions, so I have not made this an issue. For me, when sessions took longer than ninety minutes, I considered that my prerogative and did not require additional payment. However, you must come to your own determination on these issues based on the realities and practicalities of your own practice situation. Having a good rationale for your policies around fees, and conveying them clearly in advance—rather than putting too much focus on payment—paradoxically makes payment less of an issue as the healing relationship proceeds.

The other side of being clear about your fees is providing your clients ways to assess the value of your services. With energy work, progress is measured by more than just subjective feelings or even the elimination of symptoms. You can teach clients to recognize and track progress (and plateaus and setbacks) by clearly demonstrating and describing your own assessments of changes in their energies from one session to the next. You are also well advised to educate your clients about the up-and-down path healing may take, the role of healing crises, and the place of plateaus in allowing the body to rest and regroup.

CASE VIGNETTE 41

A twenty-two-year-old woman who has been responding well in your sessions quite abruptly becomes depressed for no identifiable external cause. Work with homolateral repatterning, neurovasculars, triple warmer, and stomach meridian yields only temporary relief after three intensive sessions focusing on the depression. Are you obligated at this point to refer to a mental health professional for a psychiatric assessment of the depression?

Thinking It Through

The woman had been making good progress toward her goals in working with you when symptoms of a possible psychiatric disorder emerged. You shifted your attention to the possible energetic underpinnings of her depression but have seen no lasting improvement. Relevant ethical guidelines include:

1. You perform only those services for which you are qualified, representing your education, certifications, professional affiliations, and other qualifications accurately. *(Ethics Code Highlights—6)*

2. You do not diagnose or treat illness unless you are simultaneously credentialed in a health discipline that allows you to do so. *(Competence and Scope of Practice—5)*

3. You take reasonable precautions to ensure that your personal biases, the boundaries of your competence, and the limitations of your expertise do not negatively impact the services you provide to your clients. *(General Principles—6)*

4. You know your limitations, as an individual and as a practitioner, and set your boundaries accordingly with those you serve. *(Personal Healing and Development—4)*

5. You provide services only in areas in which you have received education, training, supervised experience, or other study that qualifies you for providing those services. *(Competence and Scope of Practice—1)*

6. You assess the body's energies and energy systems, and balance and influence those energies for the client's benefit. You do not diagnose or treat illness unless simultaneously credentialed in a health discipline that allows you to do so. *(Competence and Scope of Practice—5)*

The depression may have taken the case outside your training and scope of practice. Severe depression (as well as bipolar disorder, another possibility given the progression of the case) is a potentially life-threatening illness. When the energy interventions available to you for addressing depression do not lead to improvement, you might consult an energy healing practitioner who has more experience in working with depression (numerous energy healing practitioners are simultaneously licensed in the mental health field). If you have concerns about suicide, immediate action is required, including steps to ensure her safety. In most states, when suicide is a concern, you are legally authorized to break confidentiality to protect your client and to get appropriate mental health professionals involved. Your informed consent statement should make this clear with language such as "If you make a specific threat to harm another person or yourself, I am required to communicate this to appropriate authorities."

Assuming suicidal behavior is not an immediate concern, a consultation might include discussion of issues such as your responsibilities regarding your client's depression, the methods you have already applied, what you observed after applying them, other energy healing methods that might be indicated, and considerations regarding making a referral.

In the next session with your client, you would present to her what is appropriate from the consultation. If the depression has persisted, it is time to reexamine her treatment goals in light of the new situation and to reassess whether you are the most appropriate health-care provider. As always, proceed with her health and welfare as your highest priority, speak and listen respectfully, and come to a mutually agreeable plan.

CASE VIGNETTE 42

You are invited to teach in another community. While there, your students complain that an energy healing practitioner who has previously taught in the area did not stay within the announced topic of "energy medicine" and actually taught some "far out" material that a few people liked, but many of the health providers attending felt was unfounded and inappropriate. They ultimately left with a negative impression of energy medicine. You and the other practitioner are part of the same professional association. How do you handle these complaints?

Thinking It Through

You hear complaints about a class in which you were not involved. Ethical guidelines include:

1. You assist clients, students, and the general public in developing informed judgments concerning the role of energy healing in choices that impact their health and optimal functioning. *(Public Statements and Advertising—1)*

2. If you believe there may have been an ethical violation by another energy healing practitioner, you attempt to resolve the issue by bringing it to the attention of that individual if an informal resolution appears possible and appropriate. If the issue is not adequately resolved in that fashion, you take further action appropriate to the circumstances. Such action might include informing the appropriate ethics committee of the situation. *(The Resolution of Ethical Issues—1, 2)*

3. Energy healing practitioners are responsible for their educational programs and take reasonable steps to ensure that these programs are designed to provide the appropriate knowledge and proper experiences, and to fulfill the goals of the program. *(Teaching and Presentations—1)*

4. Energy healing practitioners responsible for educational programs or presentations take reasonable steps to ensure the ready availability of accurate descriptions of the program content, goals, benefits, costs, prerequisites, and any special requirements that must be met for satisfactory completion of the program. *(Teaching and Presentations—2)*

5. Energy healing presenters anticipate the capabilities and limitations of those they teach and structure their presentations to accommodate these capabilities and limitations. *(Teaching and Presentations—3)*

6. Energy healing practitioners open themselves to feedback offered by students, clients, colleagues, and mentors. *(Personal Healing and Development—5)*

7. The integration of other modalities into an energy healing practice is allowed and encouraged, based on the energy healing practitioner's training in these modalities and best professional judgment. *(Competence and Scope of Practice—7)*

The practitioner may have breached energy healing ethics and, like it or not, you are involved by virtue of the complaints being directed toward you. This does not, however, mean that it is your responsibility to resolve the issue, or even pass judgment on the merits of the complaints, but some action is required of you. First, you need more information. Listen carefully to what the individuals who have approached you are saying and get as much information as you can about their stakes in the complaint and its resolution. Were they directly involved in the class? Do they feel they were harmed? Were their reputations as energy healing practitioners harmed? Is their primary motivation to be sure that others are forewarned? Do they feel steps should be taken with the class participants? You also need to find out what steps have been taken. Were the complaints brought to the practitioner? What transpired? Were they brought to the person who organized the course? What transpired?

With this information, your role might be to educate your students on the appropriate steps they should take (from trying to resolve the issue with the practitioner or class organizer all the way up to filing a formal complaint with the relevant ethics committee). Or you might choose to become more involved. If you know the practitioner in question and the two of you have a collegial relationship, you might decide to work with the students lodging the complaints to try to facilitate a resolution. This does put you on somewhat shaky ground, however, as the information you have is, for you, hearsay, and there might also be confidentiality issues with the people who are making the complaints not wanting to be identified. To the extent that those who were directly involved are willing and capable of moving the matter forward on their own, this should be encouraged.

You also need to be prepared to address unresolved issues from the previous class that could surface during your class. Someone might say, to use an absurd example, something like: "In the last energy medicine class I attended, we were shown how to use crystals to bend spoons, but I've just not been able to get the hang of it. Can you show me what I am doing wrong?" Though you could easily brush off such a question as not being relevant to the class you are teaching, you could also use it as an opportunity to elicit people's feelings about the last class, to respond to them sensitively, and to bring a perspective to the situation that is informative and healing. Sometimes you find yourself in a position to be part of the healing after a community rift. You are well advised to proceed cautiously and not be thrown off the announced topic of your class. There is, however, no ethical obligation to take on healing the rift, or to avoid taking it on.

CASE VIGNETTE 43

After a powerful first session, your very ill client describes the session to her minister and calls you to cancel further sessions unless you can assure her that the healing is coming from Jesus and is not the devil working through you. You sense that she is feeling very vulnerable, with her own healing at stake, and caught between two authorities. What do you do?

Thinking It Through

You are asked to claim that the results of a powerful session can be explained according to the religious framework of your client and her minister. Relevant guidelines include:

1. You consult with, refer to, or cooperate with other professionals and institutions, with your clients' consent, to the extent needed to serve the best interests of your client. *(The Healing Relationship—8)*

2. You are aware of, respect, and accommodate individual differences, including those based on religion. *(General Principles—9)*

3. You know your limitations as an individual and as a practitioner, setting your boundaries accordingly with those you serve, with colleagues, and within the larger community. *(Personal Healing and Development—4)*

4. You ensure that prospective clients understand and agree to the specifics in their informed consent form before commencing services. *(Informed Consent—2)*

5. You engage each client in identifying goals for the services being sought and mutually create an appropriate plan of care, which may include engaging other health-care professionals. *(The Healing Relationship—1)*

6. You may attempt to encourage, but do not attempt to pressure or coerce a client into any action or belief, even if you consider that such act or belief would serve the best interests of the client. *(The Healing Relationship—3)*

7. You elicit each client's expectations about energy healing and goals in using energy healing, restating them to the client for clarity and agreement, and discussing any unrealistic expectations, before providing services. Expectations are reevaluated throughout the professional relationship at times you deem appropriate. *(The Healing Relationship—5)*

8. You recognize that clear, compassionate communication is integral to providing the highest level of service possible and act accordingly. *(Personal and Interpersonal Boundaries—3)*

The first step is to ask her how she understands what occurred in the session with you and to listen to her very carefully.

Your own religious and spiritual beliefs come into play here. Even if you are not of the same religious persuasion as the woman and her minister, you may believe that there is a Force in the universe that can be elicited when believers invoke the name of Jesus, that this Force can be activated for healing, and you might have no trouble in truthfully saying some version (tailored to the situation) of: "When the name and image of Jesus were invoked in your mind, that Power came in to assist in your healing. No doubt about it!" This is certainly the path of least resistance. If it is a plausible reply for you, even if not the way you would typically frame what occurred, you might choose it since the woman's health and welfare are your highest priority and this will allow this very ill woman to continue to receive healing work that apparently has been quite beneficial.

On the other hand, if you rolled your eyes when you read this solution, it might not be quite right for you. Taking an opposite tack, you could demystify the healing work by explaining how moving the body's energies and changing the state of its electromagnetic fields using straightforward physical procedures often has a similar effect as medication, bringing about changes in molecules, cells, and organs, shifting neural pathways, and activating the immune system. The devil was not invited and did not participate. If prescription drugs from the pharmacy help her, she doesn't march into the pharmacy and demand assurance that it was not the devil.

If you go for this more scientific explanation, you have the challenge of how to get beyond the request to assure her that the healing came from

Jesus. If she will not return for another visit or even speak with you further on the phone without assurance that Jesus brought about her intense healing experience, that is her choice and is to be respected.

If, however, it is hard for you to leave it at that and you cannot resist getting yourself deeply involved, you could ask her if she would allow you to speak with her minister. If she says yes, you would, of course, need to obtain a signed release. You would engage the minister with the respect of one professional to another and try to ascertain as much as you could about what is at stake for him. Perhaps she was deliriously happy about your session with her, and he felt that any explanation other than an intervention from Jesus is inadequate. You could attempt to normalize what happened, equating it with the way a person's health improves after successful work with any physician or other competent health-care provider. Or perhaps her excitement about her session with you threatened the minister and his perceived role as the important healing force in her life. In that case, you are in a challenging situation, but you might assuage his worries by inquiring more about his faith and how he understands what happened during the session.

If you do not provide the assurance she has requested—that it was Jesus who brought about the healing—if you make no headway with the minister, and if she schedules an appointment nonetheless, you have an opportunity to speak with her frankly about how you understand the work that you do, to distinguish what you do have and do not have to offer, to explore her feelings about her minister's request and her understanding of the work she is doing with you, and to participate with her in formulating the next steps. If she decides at any point along the way to terminate services, you should respect her decision while leaving it open for her to return for further sessions.

CASE VIGNETTE 44

You use a product that has given you tremendous health benefits. You feel so strongly about it that you want to make it available to others. Is it ethical for you to sell this product to your clients? If you do not personally sell the product, is it ethical to energy test whether or not your client should use this product?

Thinking It Through

You believe this product is a major breakthrough in health care and want to make it known and available to clients who are coming to you for energy healing sessions. Relevant guidelines include:

1. You may recommend nutritional supplements, technological devices, or other healing aids only when you have adequate and appropriate knowledge to make such recommendations responsibly. *(The Healing Relationship—17)*

2. You take steps to ensure that your personal biases do not negatively impact the services you provide to your clients. *(Personal and Interpersonal Boundaries—1)*

3. You do not enter into a dual relationship that could reasonably be expected to impair your objectivity, competence, or effectiveness in the delivery of healing services. *(Personal and Interpersonal Boundaries—13)*

4. You may attempt to encourage, but you do not attempt to pressure or coerce a client into any action or belief, even if you consider that such act or belief would serve the best interests of the client. *(The Healing Relationship—3)*

5. You recognize the pitfalls of being overly attached to the outcomes of your work and of "trying too hard." *(The Healing Relationship—6)*

6. You recognize the limitations and subjective nature of nontraditional ways of assessing the flow within a client's energy system. *(The Healing Relationship—11)*

First of all, you should be suspicious of anything that feels to you like a panacea. No drug, herb, supplement, or machine has proven itself to be a cure-all or panacea within energy healing or any other form of health care. We all get excited about new discoveries and breakthroughs, yet the duration of this excitement is almost always limited, as is the degree to which the help a product gives to one person generalizes to others.

So you need to bracket your personal enthusiasm for this product from your professional practice. It is not that you cannot mention it to someone whose health condition indicates it, but if you find yourself "selling it" or discussing it with every client or routinely energy testing everyone for it, you have fallen into the "true believer" zone and need to regain your objectivity. Your biases are affecting your professional judgment.

Let's say some months have passed, your enthusiasm has mellowed, and you have found that some people who started using the product at your recommendation did not achieve the desired results, while others did. Standing on more objective ground now, you still feel this is an unusually good health-care product.

Even so, your primary area of expertise (unless you are trained and credentialed otherwise) is in the body's energy systems. While you are allowed to recommend supplements, if you do, you are required to educate yourself about their indications, contraindications, existing research, and how they compare with other products that purport to do the same thing. Your recommendations must be informed by and, as appropriate, include this information.

Many of the considerations in vignette 19 also apply here. For instance, recommending the product to your energy healing clients if you are also selling it or have another financial stake in it would be highly suspect. Mixing commerce with energy testing is particularly unacceptable since the reliability of the test rests on the tester's disinterest in the outcome.

CASE VIGNETTE 45

An energy healing colleague is in a new relationship and asks for your advice about a dilemma that has arisen. As she begins describing the situation, you realize that her new partner is one of your clients. What should you do?

Thinking It Through

You are about to receive personal information about a client from someone who is romantically involved with the client but who does not know that the person is seeing you. Relevant guidelines include:

1. You hold as the highest priority the health and welfare of your clients. *(General Principles—1)*

2. Your client is the only person who has the right to determine who has access to information about the energy healing services he or she has

received from you, including the very question of whether the client is receiving such services from you. *(Confidentiality—1)*

3. You do not enter into dual relationships that could reasonably be expected to impair the effectiveness of your services. *(Personal and Interpersonal Boundaries—13)*

4. If conflicts occur regarding your ethical obligations, you attempt to resolve these conflicts in a responsible fashion that avoids or minimizes harm. *(The Healing Relationship—15)*

You are required to think on your feet here. If you allow your colleague to keep speaking without commenting, you will be acting as if you do not know her new paramour and you will be obtaining information under false pretenses. It might also be information that in some way could adversely impact or add awkwardness to your work with your client. And if or when she learns that you are working with him, she might rightfully feel betrayed by you for not telling her this as she was pouring her heart out to you.

But if you stop her and explain why you are stopping her, you are breaking your client's confidentiality by letting your friend know you are working with him. If you stop her and don't explain why, you have created a very awkward situation and she might legitimately expect an explanation.

If you and your colleague are not close friends, you may be able to turn the conversation gracefully away from her new relationship without undue suspicion or awkwardness. If you are close friends, accustomed to sharing personal issues, this probably won't work. You could, however, stall. You could excuse yourself, saying there is an important call you need to make, and call your client, state your dilemma (you are not bound to confidentiality that you are friends with your colleague), and inquire whether he objects to your revealing that you are seeing him as a client. If he does, discuss other possible solutions given the circumstances. If he does not object to your revealing that you are working with him professionally, you can assure him that you will reveal no other personal information. Clear boundaries have suddenly become a paramount issue in your work with this man.

If you cannot call him or reach him at that moment, you might judge the situation as being so ethically perilous that you abruptly end the meeting with a vague excuse in order to buy time to consult with your client about the situation and enlist him to tell or to give you permission to tell.

If you cannot reach the client or end the meeting, you may simply need to find a way to redirect the conversation.

CASE VIGNETTE 46

An energy healing colleague who is part of your professional association reveals that she has entered into a sexual relationship with a client. She is thrilled with this development. Are you obligated to report her to your ethics committee?

Thinking It Through

Your colleague has confided in you that she has committed a major ethical violation yet she seems unaware that her action was an ethical violation. Relevant guidelines include:

1. Dual relationships that are never acceptable are ones in which the practitioner develops any kind of romantic or sexual relationship with the client while energy healing services are being provided. *(Personal and Interpersonal Boundaries—17)*

2. Energy healing practitioners do not engage in sexual relations with a former client for at least a year after termination of the client relationship, and only then after a good faith determination through appropriate consultation that there is no exploitation of the former client. *(Personal and Interpersonal Boundaries—18)*

3. Energy healing practitioners refrain from entering into a dual relationship if the dual relationship could reasonably be expected to impair the practitioner's objectivity, competence, or effectiveness in the delivery of healing or educational services, or otherwise risks exploitation or harm to the person with whom the professional relationship exists. *(Personal and Interpersonal Boundaries—13)*

4. When energy healing practitioners believe there may have been an ethical violation by another energy healing practitioner, they attempt to resolve the issue by bringing it to the attention of that individual if an informal resolution appears possible and appropriate. If the issue is not adequately resolved in that fashion, energy healing practitioners take

further action appropriate to the circumstances. Such action might include informing the relevant ethics committee of the situation. *(The Resolution of Ethical Issues—1, 2)*

Your colleague is bound by an ethics code that prohibits entering into a sexual relationship with a client. Yet she seems totally oblivious to the fact that she has violated a fundamental standard. You may wonder, "What was she thinking?" Was this one of those situations where "the mind, even of a sincere professional health-care provider, can powerfully rationalize inappropriate behavior when driven by romantic and/or sexual desire"? Is there more to the story?

She wants you to be happy for her. But you are bound by an ethics code that compels you to take action when you are aware that a fellow practitioner has violated professional ethics. You also are aware that she has put her client's welfare in jeopardy. You hate to be the one who has to break the news to her, but that is your ethical obligation. The "Ethics Code for Energy Healing Practitioners" instructs you to "attempt to resolve the issue by bringing it to the [person's] attention if an informal resolution appears possible and appropriate." If this does not lead to an ethical resolution of the problem, you are obligated to report the situation to the appropriate ethics committee.

Out of respect for your colleague and the process, however, you might tell her, face-to-face, what you are thinking. You might begin by inquiring how she reconciles her new sexual relationship with the ethical restriction on engaging in sex with a client. Is there any mitigating circumstance that might not require you to file a report to the ethics committee? Perhaps you learn that it was all a misunderstanding: he was her client in her seamstress business, not her energy healing practice. Perhaps she terminated the professional energy healing relationship before entering a personal one and had, in consultation with a colleague, decided that the "One-Year Rule" *(Personal and Interpersonal Boundaries—18)* is an inappropriate restriction for her situation. Find out about the circumstances and whether she believes ethical issues are involved. If she knows they are, find out how she intends to handle them. In this vignette, there are few scenarios in which you would not be required to report her to an ethics committee, but you should begin your inquiry with an open mind that initially gives her the benefit of the doubt.

CASE VIGNETTE 47

An energy healing colleague reveals that she has entered into a sexual relationship with a client. She is agonizing about this development and seeking your counsel. Are you obligated to report her to the ethics committee of your professional association?

This is identical to the previous vignette, except for the crucial difference that, rather than being oblivious to the ethical violation, the practitioner is agonizing about it and seeking your counsel. In addition to all the ethical guidelines listed in the previous discussion, one more rule applies here:

"Energy healing practitioners are not obligated to take action based on information gained when serving as a member of a peer review panel, as an advisor to another practitioner who is seeking consultation on the specific ethical situation in question, or as a mediator between a practitioner and one or more clients." *(The Resolution of Ethical Issues—2, paragraph 2)*

This guideline makes space for a practitioner who has committed an ethical violation to seek counseling and to have that counseling protected by the seal of confidentiality. She is not protected, however, if other energy healing practitioners learn about the situation. But you are not obligated or, in fact, allowed to discuss her case with her ethics committee or anyone else, except if you seek supervision, which would also be sealed by confidentiality. Situations of clear and imminent physical danger or abuse of a minor, however, always override the seal of confidentiality.

Having been asked to serve as her confidante and counselor, you need to assess whether you feel confident about taking on this complex responsibility. She has created a mess and she knows it. She must now decide what steps to take that best serve her client's welfare and her own welfare, and possibly salvage her career, while managing her emotional turmoil. At the same time, she needs to be doing the self-examination that will help her find her way out of the quagmire with the least damage done and that will help keep her from repeating it. Your decision about whether to take on this enormous responsibility might not, however, need to be an all-or-nothing choice. You might, for instance, decide that you can help her think through the professional issues but insist that she enlist a trained psychotherapist to help her with the emotional dimensions of the situation.

CASE VIGNETTE 48

In working with a minor child, you suspect that there is some form of abuse currently taking place. How do you handle this with the child? If the child confirms your suspicions, what do you do then? What do you do if the person bringing the child for the appointments is the suspected abuser?

Thinking It Through

While working with a child's health concerns, you suspect that the child is being abused. Relevant guidelines include:

1. You hold as your highest priority the health and welfare of your client. (*General Principles—1*)

2. Your client (or the client's legal guardian or conservator) is the only person who has the right to determine who has access to information about the energy healing services information he or she has received from you. (*Confidentiality—1*)

3. You monitor the effects of your own mental state and ego needs on your ability to help those with whom you work. (*Personal Healing and Development—2*)

4. You recognize the pitfalls of being overly attached to the outcomes of the services you provide. (*The Healing Relationship—6*)

5. You refer to other professions and institutions to the extent needed to serve the best interests of your client. (*The Healing Relationship—8*)

6. You disclose information that would prevent clear and imminent danger to your client. (*Confidentiality—1, Exception a*)

The laws in most states are very clear that you must inform the appropriate authorities if you have a reasonable basis for suspecting that a child or a senior citizen is being physically or sexually abused. This overrides any confidentiality protection found in state laws or professional ethics. You must, in fact, be prepared to lose the client if abuse is not substantiated in an investigation.

If you do not know the laws and procedures in your state and region regarding such situations, familiarize yourself with them (for starters, you could go to *www.about.com*, enter "How to Report Child Abuse" in the search engine, go to the article by that name, peruse it, find the relevant phone number for your state, place a call, and ask for information about your state's laws and procedures). You can also anonymously call Child Protective Services, present the situation with no identifying information, and request a telephone consultation.

In this vignette, you suspect but do not know whether child abuse is occurring. The first step is to do a quick inner examination to determine if anything in the child's situation may have triggered something involving abuse from your own personal history. If you have doubts about whether your suspicions are your own projections, immediately consult with a colleague or counselor so you can maximize your objectivity in managing the situation.

The line between "wondering" and "a reasonable basis for suspecting," can be a very delicate call. Not reporting when abuse is occurring may result in continued and substantial harm to the child. Reporting when abuse is not occurring may not only cost the parties involved dearly, but also their sense of betrayal could cause the end of your healing work with the child. Discussing the evidence you do have with a colleague or supervisor might be a constructive step in coming to an appropriate determination.

Eliciting more information from the child is an option open to you. However, it is a more precarious option than might be obvious. Mental health specialists who are trained in determining whether a child has been abused not only use clear, age-appropriate language in interviewing the child, they also know how to avoid leading language or questions that might cause the child to validate their words out of confusion, a desire to please, or not knowing what else to say. If the child becomes uncomfortable or agitated, they know how to pull back on the inquiry or on its intensity. They also know how to utilize play therapy, mutual storytelling, and other less linear techniques to gather information. If you do not have such training, you are wiser to report your suspicions to the appropriate authorities even though there is a degree of uncertainty.

If you have a reasonable basis for suspecting child abuse, and the suspected abuser is outside the immediate family, you would most likely ask to have a meeting with one or both parents as soon as possible. If the suspected abuser is inside the immediate family, you would be wise to contact your local Child Protective Services agency and discuss next steps.

Generally, you should not confront the alleged abuser, at least not before contacting appropriate authorities.

Case Vignette 49

You attend a lecture in which an energy healing practitioner takes credit for other people's ideas, presenting them as her own. Is this an ethical problem? How should you handle it?

Thinking It Through

You are surprised to hear your colleague publicly claim credit for ideas that you know others developed. Relevant guidelines include:

1. Energy healing practitioners credit colleagues for their contributions and innovations and show respect for the teachings, teachers, and practitioners that went before them. *(Personal and Interpersonal Boundaries—12)*

2. Energy healing practitioners credit those whose methods or other contributions are being taught. *(Teaching and Presentations—4)*

3. Energy healing practitioners promote accuracy, honesty, and truthfulness in their communications and in the practice, teaching, science, and art of energy healing. *(General Principles—4)*

4. If you believe there may have been an ethical violation by another energy healing practitioner, you attempt to resolve the issue by bringing it to the attention of that individual if an informal resolution appears possible and appropriate. If the issue is not adequately resolved in that fashion, you take further action appropriate to the circumstances. Such action might include informing the relevant ethics committee of the situation. *(The Resolution of Ethical Issues—1, 2)*

The circumstances dictate some of your options. If you are able to chat with the lecturer during a break, you could present your concern and the lecturer would have an opportunity to agree and correct the misstatements in the group's presence, to disagree and perhaps present you with information about which you were not aware that supports the statements that were made from the stage, or to receive the information from you but do nothing with it. If the misstatements are corrected from the stage, or if you are shown that you were incorrect about who deserves credit for the ideas, the ethical issue is resolved.

If your concerns are accurate and the lecturer does nothing about the situation, or if you are only able to present your concerns after the lecture and you have a chance to validate them, further action is necessary.

If the lecturer owns having made a mistake, you could explore reasonable actions. For instance, if the e-mail addresses of those who attended the lecture are available, a note correcting the misstatements could be sent out. At a minimum, in terms of an ethical resolution, if it is not possible or practical to contact those who attended the lecture, the lecturer would agree to abstain from making the misstatements in the future and would agree to correct any handouts that contained the misstatements.

If the lecturer is defensive or angry about the feedback you have offered, is not able to provide any information to the contrary, and is unwilling to consider any corrective action, you could escalate the feedback to a discussion of an ethical violation. In almost all probable scenarios arising from this vignette, a resolution would be reached before that, but a complaint to the appropriate ethics committee would be available to you as a last resort.

CASE VIGNETTE 50

You have a female client who loves dogs and dog shows. She's a wonderful person who would love to be in a relationship. You have another client who shows his dogs regularly and is also single. You're sure they would be great for each other. What do you do?

Thinking It Through

You are working with two single clients who share a common interest and you sense they would be romantically interested in one another if you were able to introduce them. Relevant guidelines include:

1. You recognize the pitfalls of becoming overly attached, "trying too hard," or micromanaging a client. (*The Healing Relationship—6*)

2. You take reasonable precautions to ensure that your personal biases do not negatively impact the services you provide to your clients. (*Personal and Interpersonal Boundaries—1*)

3. You are sensitive to differences in power between yourself as a caregiver and your clients and do not exploit such differences. *(Personal and Interpersonal Boundaries—10)*

4. You do not enter into a dual relationship if the dual relationship could reasonably be expected to impair your objectivity or effectiveness in the delivery of healing services or otherwise risks exploitation or harm to the person with whom the professional relationship exists. *(Personal and Interpersonal Boundaries—13)*

5. You respect the rights of individuals to self-determination. (*General Principles—7*)

6. Your client is the only person who has the right to determine who has access to information about the energy healing services he or she has received from you, including the very question of whether the client is receiving such services from you. *(Confidentiality—1)*

You are tempted to act as Cupid for two people who are single and whose potential compatibility seems likely. But even if you are an incurable romantic and very proud of your track record for matchmaking, the professional relationships place constraints on this situation. The purpose of your relationship with these two people is to apply an energy approach to enhance their health. In that role, you are viewed as an authority about highly personal matters. That is why you are being paid. If you convey your fantasy that the two of them might be a good match, you are exerting your authority beyond the scope of your professional competence. Though this might seem a subtle distinction to you, it could have strong reverberations. If you do, in one way or another, get them together, their choices in the early stages of the relationship may well be influenced by echoes of your encouragement rather than their own perceptions and self-determination. What started for you as a kind of sentimental musing might translate into greater influence than you ever imagined or would want.

Besides propelling the relationship with the wrong fuel, stepping in as matchmaker might also negatively impact your professional relationship with one or both clients. What if the romance starts strongly but quickly cools off for one, and the other is left in a heap? The one who lost interest might wonder, "What were you thinking?" while the one who was hurt might focus the sessions on healing the wound, with an underlying theme of having been betrayed by you and by your other client. In any case, the act of matchmaking crosses professional boundaries in ways that energetically compromise the healing relationship and may compromise it in more tangible ways as well. Keep your focus on optimizing your clients' energies and leave it to them to figure out what to do with those enhanced energies. And leave matchmaking to friends and family. Their good intentions can create enough havoc in your clients' lives.

CHAPTER 4

Ethics Code for Energy Healing Practitioners

Ethical standards include the highest ethical ideals of a profession, serving to ennoble and inspire practitioners, and also enforce obligations regarding acceptable practice. Ethical standards inform all of a practitioner's professional activities and include specific responsibilities to clients. You are free to choose whom you admit as a client. Once you accept a person as a client, however, you have a duty to provide appropriate health-care services or, when you cannot, to offer appropriate referrals to ensure the best possible health-care services.

Lack of awareness or understanding of a stated ethical standard is not a valid defense against a charge of unethical conduct. Because it is not possible to write an exhaustive ethics code that covers every conceivable situation, circumstances not specifically addressed here may still be evaluated in terms of ethical conduct.

I. General Principles

1. Energy healing (EH) practitioners hold as the highest priority for their professional activities the health and welfare of their clients, students, and others with whom they become professionally involved. All other statements in this document are elaborations upon this principle.

2. EH practitioners are committed to a lifelong process of personal development in body, mind, and spirit.

3. EH practitioners uphold professional standards of conduct and accept appropriate responsibility for their own behavior.

4. EH practitioners promote accuracy, honesty, and truthfulness in their communications and in the practice, teaching, science, and art of energy healing.

5. EH practitioners keep their agreements and avoid unrealistic or unclear commitments.

6. EH practitioners take reasonable[3] precautions to ensure that their personal biases, the boundaries of their competence, impairments to their health and well-being, and the limitations of their expertise do not negatively impact the services they provide to their clients.

7. EH practitioners respect the dignity, worth, and uniqueness of all people, and the rights of individuals to privacy, confidentiality, and self-determination.

8. EH practitioners are committed to giving all persons access to and benefit from the contributions of energy healing, while retaining the right to maintain their integrity, best judgment, and personal safety at all times.

9. EH practitioners are aware of, respect, and accommodate individual, cultural, and role differences, including those based on age, gender, gender identity, race, ethnicity, culture, national origin, religion, sexual orientation, disability, language, representational system, element, and socioeconomic status.

10. EH practitioners contribute a portion of their professional time for little or no compensation.

11. EH practitioners demonstrate a personal commitment to acting ethically; modeling ethical behavior, encouraging ethical behavior by students, supervisees, employees, and colleagues; and consulting with others concerning ethical problems.

---

3 As used in this ethics statement, the term *reasonable* means the prevailing professional judgment of health practitioners engaged in similar activities in similar circumstances, given the knowledge the practitioner had or should have had at the time. It is used here to ensure applicability across a broad range of contexts and to guard against establishing a set of rigid rules that might be applied out of context.

II. Personal Healing and Development

Energy healing is, by nature, a holistic approach to well-being in that energy interacts seamlessly with mind, body, and spirit. Practitioners recognize that EH involves a way of relating to life as well as mastery of a particular set of concepts and techniques. With that consciousness, EH practitioners are committed to their own ongoing healing and the wholesome development of body, mind, and spirit.

The more practitioners have evolved personally through activities that promote awareness, health, and healing, the more proficient they become as healers and the more likely they will be to behave competently, responsibly, and ethically with those entrusted to their care, with their colleagues, and with the wider community. In the same sense that health is more than the absence of illness, self-awareness involves a commitment to discover and go beyond limitations in one's understanding and perspective, such as those rooted in unprocessed trauma or personal or professional insecurities that could have a negative impact on professional activities.

EH practitioners are aware that their personal limitations can have direct impact on the quality of the services they provide to clients and students. They are equally aware that the skills they develop in their own quest for wholeness can contribute not only to their personal development, but to their professional development as well. The obligation to cultivate personal growth and awareness, because of its impact on the quality of service a practitioner is able to provide, is an essential, ongoing process.

1. EH practitioners are committed to maintaining a personal program of their own design for developing body, mind, and spirit.

2. EH practitioners monitor the effects of their own physical health, mental state, and ego needs on their ability to help those with whom they work and take appropriate steps to maximize their well-being in each area.

3. EH practitioners have personally experienced the methods they offer others, using their own experiences with EH as a laboratory for further informing themselves about the value and power of specific techniques. At the same time, they take care not to project their experiences with a particular method onto others.

4. EH practitioners know their limitations as individuals and as practitioners, setting their boundaries accordingly with those they serve, with colleagues, and within the larger community.

5. EH practitioners open themselves to feedback offered by their students, clients, colleagues, and mentors.

6. EH practitioners closely monitor their needs to be liked, to be admired, to achieve status, and to exercise power, as well as their sexual and romantic needs, and seek feedback, guidance, consultation, and supervision from friends, colleagues, mentors, supervisors, or other professionals to keep these needs from interfering with their effectiveness in the services they provide.

7. EH Practitioners examine their professional association's ethics code in the context of their own religious and spiritual beliefs or other personal codes of conduct, and address any conflicts with officials in their professional association.

III. Competence and Scope of Practice

1. EH practitioners provide health care, education, supervision, consultation, and mentoring services only in areas in which they have received education, training, supervised experience, or other study that qualifies them for providing those services. For instance, while coursework in energy psychology might give an energy medicine practitioner tools for teaching some basic techniques for emotional self-management, it does not qualify a practitioner to provide psychotherapy. It is the responsibility of the practitioner to draw those lines professionally and appropriately.

2. EH practitioners provide information to prospective clients about their background in both EH and other modalities that may be used. This information should address the limitations of their training regarding issues such as the diagnosis and treatment of illness, possible side effects, and the fact that energy medicine and energy psychology are considered unconventional approaches to health care.

3. EH practitioners stay current in their field of practice and maintain and further develop their competence on an ongoing basis through

supervision, consultations, workshops, published works, electronic media, and continuing education courses.

4. EH practitioners obtain appropriate insurance, permits, and licenses, and they comply with other sound business practices.

5. EH practitioners assess the body's energies and energy systems, and balance and influence those energies for the client's benefit. They do not *diagnose* or *treat* illness unless they are simultaneously credentialed in a health discipline that allows them to do so.[4]

6. EH practitioners working with severe trauma have received appropriate training.

7. The integration of other modalities into an EH practice is allowed and encouraged, based on the practitioner's training in these modalities and best professional judgment.

8. EH practitioners take steps to promote their own cultural sensitivity and their awareness of the special needs of vulnerable populations such as prisoners, children, the elderly, and the mentally or physically impaired.

9. When EH practitioners provide services in emergency situations, they may use their best professional judgment in going beyond their usual scope of practice when health-care practitioners who are more fully qualified to provide needed interventions are not available. Beyond appropriate follow-up, they discontinue these services, in a spirit of respect and cooperation, when the emergency has ended or more appropriate services are available.

IV. Informed Consent

1. EH practitioners utilize a signed "informed consent" form or other device (such as discussion of specific issues, recorded in the client's

---

4 Some EH practitioners are licensed, certified, or otherwise recognized in, and simultaneously practice, other healing modalities. The "Ethics Code for Energy Healing Practitioners" presupposes that EH practitioners who are bound to another code of ethics and standards of practice by virtue of their licensure and/or membership in an organization of their fellow professionals will integrate the "Ethics Code for Energy Healing Practitioners" with their own profession's codes and standards.

case notes) to provide clear information to prospective clients about the nature of their services and the logistics of their practice (including but not limited to length and frequency of sessions, fees, cancellation policies, the nature of assessment and care, etc.).

2. EH practitioners understand that informed consent begins with their website and other advertising.

3. EH practitioners ensure that prospective clients understand and agree to the specifics in their informed consent form before commencing EH services.

4. In deciding whether to provide services to those already receiving health services elsewhere, EH practitioners carefully consider the health-care issues and the prospective client's welfare. They discuss these issues with the client (or a legally authorized person on behalf of the client) in order to minimize the risk of confusion and conflict, consult with the other service providers when appropriate, and, in a spirit of respect and cooperation toward all related parties, proceed with sensitivity to the health-care issues involved.

V. The Healing Relationship

1. EH practitioners engage each client in identifying goals for the services being sought and in mutually creating a suitable plan of care, which may, as appropriate, include engaging other health-care professionals.

2. EH clients are encouraged to be proactive about their own health needs and to take responsibility for their health-care choices.

3. EH practitioners may attempt to encourage, but they do not attempt to pressure or coerce a client into any action or belief, even if the practitioner considers that such act or belief would serve the best interests of the client.

4. Though it is appropriate to encourage hope and convey confidence in EH methods, EH practitioners do so without overstating the power of the methods or implying that a method that has helped some people with a particular health issue will help all people with that issue. They also proceed with sensitivity in order to abstain from fostering guilt in clients who are not responding as hoped.

5. EH practitioners not only elicit each client's hopes and expectations for using EH, they also discuss any unrealistic expectations as early in the healing relationship as is reasonable. Expectations are reevaluated throughout the professional relationship at times deemed appropriate by the practitioner or at any time at the client's request.

6. EH practitioners recognize the pitfalls of being overly attached to the outcomes of the services they provide. "Trying too hard," micromanaging a client, or becoming overly invested may have a paradoxical effect. This is one of the dilemmas that should be considered before providing health-care services to family or friends.

7. EH practitioners exercise the right to refuse to accept into their care any person seeking their services when they judge this not to be in the best interests of the client or a threat to their own personal safety.

8. EH practitioners consult with, refer to, or cooperate with other professionals and institutions, with their clients' consent, to the extent needed to serve the best interests of their clients. In particular, they understand the boundaries and limitations of their services and make referrals accordingly. They are clear with clients about whether or not they have personal knowledge of the skills of a particular practitioner and encourage clients to interview prospective practitioners before committing themselves to that practitioner's care.

9. EH practitioners provide a safe, clean, welcoming, supportive, appropriate, and comfortable environment for their services that is conducive to healing. They also provide their undivided and uninterrupted attention during an EH session.

10. EH practitioners recognize and articulate what is healthy and right in the person's energies as well as identify areas requiring attention.

11. EH practitioners may use "energy testing" and other nontraditional ways of assessing the flow within a client's energy system. They understand, however, the limitations and subjective nature of such methods. EH practitioners realize that energy testing is intended to assess the body's energies and is not to be used to replace physical diagnostic tests or to confirm or invalidate beliefs, memories, or anticipated courses of action. EH practitioners are particularly cautious about energy testing potential customers on products they are selling.

12. EH shall always be administered in a caring, considerate manner, with respect for the client's preferences and capacities. Clients shall be informed in advance about the purpose of any invasive procedures and given an explicit choice about whether to proceed or to have alternative methods applied. If the choice is to proceed, agreement is reached in advance about how the client will communicate to the practitioner the desire to stop the procedure. The practitioner will instantly respect this signal and immediately halt the procedures.

13. EH practitioners are sensitive to a client's feelings about being touched, discuss those feelings, as appropriate, and gain permission before applying any procedure that requires touch. For procedures that require making contact or putting pressure in the areas of a client's genitals, breasts, buttocks, navel, or throat, the practitioner is especially alert to the client's sensitivities and offers alternative methods, if appropriate, such as asking clients to use their own hands for making the direct contact.

14. If limitations to services can be anticipated because of financial hardship, the related issues are discussed with the recipient of services as early as is feasible. EH practitioners do not maintain a client relationship solely for financial reasons, but they may terminate a relationship if the client is unable or unwilling to pay for such services. Prior to any termination of services, the issues involved and possible alternatives are discussed, with the client's well-being as the highest priority.

15. If conflicts occur regarding EH practitioners' ethical obligations, EH practitioners attempt to resolve these conflicts in a responsible fashion that avoids or minimizes harm, seeking consultation or supervision as appropriate.

16. EH practitioners may choose to barter[5] for services only if this arrangement will not interfere with the quality of the services being provided and if the resulting arrangement is not exploitative to either party.

17. EH practitioners may recommend nutritional supplements, technological devices, or other healing aids only when they have adequate and appropriate qualifications to make such recommendations responsibly.

---

5 Barter is the acceptance of goods, services, or other nonmonetary remuneration from clients in return for EH services.

18 EH practitioners terminate a client relationship when it becomes reasonably clear that the client no longer needs or is no longer benefiting from the continued service.

19. EH practitioners who reach an interpersonal impasse with a client or a dead end in the healing services they are providing consider a range of options, such as enlisting supervision, suggesting bringing a consultant into a session, referring the client to another practitioner, or suggesting terminating their services.

20. EH practitioners may terminate a client relationship if they feel their physical safety is at risk.

21. Practitioners who are in an ongoing relationship providing EH services make reasonable efforts to facilitate a continuity of services in the event that their services are interrupted by factors such as their illness, relocation, retirement, or by the client's relocation or financial limitations.

22. Responsibilities of the EH practitioner following termination of services include continuing to maintain confidentiality and sharing client information with other professionals as requested by the client. If the client requests that such information be forwarded, it may not be withheld for any reason, including nonpayment of fees.

VI. Confidentiality

1. The client (or the client's legal guardian or conservator) is the only person who has the right to determine who has access to information about the EH services the client receives, including the very question of whether the client is receiving such services from the practitioner. Exceptions to this principle are made explicit in the disclosure statements:

    a. *Exception:* When disclosure of information is required to prevent clear and imminent danger to the client or to others.

    b. *Exception:* When there is a clear legal requirement in the country, region, or area to disclose certain types of information.

    c. *Exception:* When records are subpoenaed by a court.

    d. *Exception:* If the EH practitioner is a defendant in a civil, criminal, or disciplinary action arising from the client relationship, information about that relationship may be disclosed as part of the proceeding.

e. ***Exception:*** EH practitioners who seek *consultation* or *supervisory* services from other EH practitioners agree that information about their competency may be disclosed to designated professional associations (with client identity concealed) for the purpose of evaluating the practitioner's readiness to enter advanced training or to be listed for referral.

2. EH practitioners who work with children or with more than one member of the same family (including "significant others") establish with the relevant parties at the outset (or when new family members begin to receive services from the practitioner) the kinds of information that may be shared, and with whom, and the kinds of information that may not be shared by the practitioner. Services are provided to more than one member of a family only after weighing potential disadvantages, conflicts, and confidentiality issues.

3. When consulting with colleagues, EH practitioners do not disclose confidential information that could reasonably lead to the identification of a client with whom they have a confidential relationship unless they have obtained the prior consent of the person or the disclosure cannot be avoided. Informed consent forms may include a stipulation that the practitioner can seek supervision or consultation about the client.

4. Before recording the voices or images of individuals to whom they provide services, EH practitioners obtain permission from all such persons or their legal representatives and disclose how the voices or images may be used.

5. EH practitioners do not disclose in their writings, lectures, or other public media personally identifiable information concerning their clients, students, research participants, or other recipients of their services that they obtained during the course of their work unless (1) they take reasonable steps to disguise the recipient of service, (2) the recipient has consented in writing or in the recorded session, or (3) there is legal authorization for doing so.

VII. Personal and Interpersonal Boundaries

1. EH practitioners take steps to ensure that their personal biases, the boundaries of their competence, and the limitations of their training do not negatively impact the services they provide to their clients.

2. EH practitioners clarify professional roles and obligations and seek to manage conflicts of interest to avoid exploitation or harm.

3. EH practitioners recognize that clear, compassionate communication is integral to providing the highest level of service possible and act accordingly.

4. EH services may open issues that are private, delicate, or embarrassing. EH practitioners are prepared to articulate these issues when they emerge and discuss them in a frank, professional, and respectful manner, while at the same time acknowledging the client's right not to discuss the issue.

5. EH practitioners recognize that, in dealing directly with their client's energy systems, the subtle nature of those energy systems and their sometimes intangible perception can at times create boundary issues that don't arise in other disciplines. EH practitioners maintain appropriate boundaries, acknowledge the client's authority to make fundamental choices about the healing relationship, and recognize how the wisdom of the client's body also directs the healing process. EH practitioners do not aggrandize themselves or dramatize their abilities to perceive or work with subtle energies.

6. EH practitioners do not use their abilities to work with energy to wield power over another person, to manipulate another person, or to create an unequal relationship with another person. This includes, but is not limited to, abilities associated with intuition or other intangible means of assessment.

7. Because EH practitioners work with their clients' energies, they acknowledge a special responsibility to take steps that keep their own energy systems strong and resilient, and they utilize methods that decrease their vulnerability to being negatively impacted by the energies of their clients.

8. If an EH practitioner is unable to offer services competently due to illness, stress, or other factors, or if personal problems are likely to

interfere with competently performing a professional activity, the practitioner cancels or postpones the activity until the limiting factors have been resolved.

9. EH practitioners do not provide services under the influence of any medication, drug, other substance, or state of mind that might impair their work.

10. EH practitioners are sensitive to differences in power between the practitioner and the client and do not exploit such differences during or after the professional relationship for the benefit or personal gratification of the practitioner.

11. EH practitioners obtain explicit or clearly implied permission prior to engaging in "distant," "remote," "surrogate," or "nonlocal" assessment or healing, and they perform such services with the client's welfare as their highest priority.

12. EH practitioners treat colleagues with dignity, respect, and courtesy; talk about colleagues in respectful ways; resist gossip; credit colleagues for their contributions and innovations; and show respect for the teachings, teachers, and practitioners before them.

13. EH practitioners do not enter into a dual relationship[6] that could reasonably be expected to impair the practitioner's objectivity, competence, or effectiveness in the delivery of healing or educational services, or otherwise risks exploitation or harm to the person with whom the professional relationship exists.

14. Dual relationships that would not reasonably be expected to cause impairment or risk exploitation or harm are not unethical. However, it is the practitioner's responsibility to ensure that each party is aware of issues related to shifting between the client-practitioner setting and the social setting of the personal relationship. These issues should be discussed with the client and take precedence in decisions about the dual relationship.

---

6 A dual relationship occurs when an EH practitioner is in a professional role with a person and 1) at the same time is in another role with the same person, 2) at the same time is in a relationship with a person closely associated with or related to the person with whom the practitioner has the professional relationship, or 3) promises to enter into another role in the future with the person or a person closely associated with or related to the person.

15. If an EH practitioner finds that, due to unforeseen factors, a potentially harmful dual relationship has arisen, the practitioner takes reasonable steps to resolve it with due regard for the best interests of the affected person and maximal compliance with the "Ethics Code for Energy Healing Practitioners."

16. When EH practitioners are required by law, institutional policy, or extraordinary circumstances to serve in more than one role in judicial or administrative proceedings, they clarify role expectations and the extent of confidentiality as early as possible.

17. Dual relationships that are never acceptable are ones in which a practitioner develops any kind of romantic or sexual relationship with any client while EH services are being provided.

18. EH practitioners do not engage in sexual relations with a former client for at least a full year after termination of the client relationship, and only then after a good faith determination through appropriate consultation that there is no exploitation of the former client.

19. In their work-related activities, EH practitioners model respect and tolerance and do not engage in harassment or demeaning behavior toward others or unfair discrimination based on age, gender, gender identity, race, ethnicity, culture, national origin, religion, sexual orientation, disability, or socioeconomic status. EH practitioners do, however, reserve the right to refuse service to anyone they feel may compromise their safety.

20. EH practitioners do not engage in sexual harassment. Sexual harassment includes sexual solicitation, physical advances, energetic advances, or verbal or nonverbal conduct that is sexual in nature, that occurs in connection with the practitioner's professional role or activities, and that is: (1) unwelcome, offensive, or creates an objectionable interpersonal atmosphere and the practitioner has been informed of this; (2) sufficiently severe or intense to be considered abusive to a reasonable person in the same context; or (3) unnecessarily or inappropriately provocative under the guise of evaluating a health concern or providing services. Sexual harassment can consist of a single severe act or of persistent multiple acts of less intensity. This principle applies in all professional settings, from the consulting room to the classroom.

VIII. Record Keeping

1. EH practitioners document having acquired informed consent from all clients.

2. EH practitioners use their own professional judgment on the kinds of intake information, assessments, interventions, and session-by-session outcomes they record and maintain in the client's file.

3. EH practitioners store client records in a safe and secure place, maintain such records for at least seven years (or longer if dictated by legal requirements or other circumstances) following the termination of services, and dispose of client records in a secure manner.

4. EH practitioners do not alter records. Additions that correct earlier information should be dated.

5. EH practitioners ensure that clerical or other staff members who have access to client records are educated to do so only under strictly controlled circumstances and to uphold confidentiality at all times.

6. EH practitioners adhere to the principle that any client records to be used for research purposes may be used only with the client's written consent or with pertinent identifying personal information removed or adequately disguised.

7. EH practitioners maintain session records, if they are licensed in an allied profession, in the manner required by that particular profession.

8. EH practitioners are aware of and adhere to relevant laws and regulations regarding a client's right to obtain his or her EH records.

IX. Public Statements and Advertising

1. EH practitioners assist clients, students, and the general public in developing informed judgments concerning the role of energy healing in choices that impact their health and optimal functioning.

2. Public statements, whether intended for informational or advertising purposes, should be evaluated for any unintended impact before they are released.

3. EH practitioners use clear, accessible language in their advertisements, and their advertisements are honest, dignified, and representative of services that can be delivered.

4. EH practitioners do not make false, deceptive, or fraudulent statements concerning: (1) their training, experience, or competence; (2) their academic degrees; (3) their credentials; (4) their institutional or association affiliations; (5) their services; (6) the scientific or clinical basis for, results of, or degree of success of their services; (7) their fees; or (8) their publications or research findings.

5. EH practitioners do not make public statements that use sensationalism or that prey on the public's vulnerability to irrational fears and anxieties.

6. EH practitioners who engage others to create or place public statements that promote their professional practice, products, or activities retain professional responsibility for such statements.

7. EH practitioners do not compensate employees of press, radio, television, or other communication media in return for publicity in a news item.

8. EH practitioners associated with the development or promotion of products disclose any vested interest when informing clients or students about such products and ensure that such products are presented in a factual and professional manner.

9. A paid advertisement relating to an EH practitioner's activities or products must be identified or clearly recognizable as such.

10. To the degree to which they exercise control, EH practitioners responsible for announcements, catalogs, brochures, or advertisements describing workshops, seminars, or other educational programs ensure that they accurately describe the audience for which the program is intended, the educational objectives, the presenters, and the fees involved.

11. When EH practitioners provide public advice or comment via radio, television, print, or Internet, they take precautions to ensure that statements are based on their professional knowledge, training, or experience and that the welfare of any demonstration subjects is of highest priority.

12. If EH practitioners learn of the misuse or misrepresentation of their work, they take reasonable steps to correct or minimize the misuse or misrepresentation.

X. Teaching and Presentations

1. **EH** practitioners responsible for educational programs or presentations take reasonable steps to ensure that the programs are designed to provide the appropriate knowledge and proper experiences and to fulfill the goals of the presentation or program. This may require that the practitioner has acquired experience or training in curriculum design and presentation methods.

2. EH practitioners responsible for educational programs or presentations take reasonable steps to ensure the ready availability of accurate descriptions of the program content, goals, benefits, costs, prerequisites, and any special requirements that must be met for satisfactory completion of the program.

3. EH teachers anticipate the capabilities and limitations of those they teach and structure their presentations to accommodate these capabilities and limitations.

4. EH teachers appropriately credit those whose methods, theories, research, or other contributions are being taught.

5. EH teachers convey the appropriate applications of the methods and concepts being presented, including their limitations and any risks.

6. EH teachers develop methods to evaluate the proficiency of those they train prior to providing any formal certification of competency.

7. EH teachers prioritize the welfare of volunteers for demonstrations above the presentation itself, taking all reasonable steps to ensure that volunteers who are selected for demonstrations will not be harmed by the demonstration.

8. EH teachers provide follow-up for any immediate distress that arises during or as a consequence of a demonstration and offer an appropriate referral. They do not charge for such follow-up in this circumstance.

9. If a more serious health issue is uncovered during a demonstration, or if what is uncovered goes beyond the scope of the demonstration, the

presenter is not obligated to provide ongoing services to resolve that issue. The presenter's obligation is limited to providing immediate first aid, as described in #8, and referral suggestions.

10. EH teachers who show video or audiotapes of their work are responsible for acquiring the informed consent of those portrayed.

11. EH practitioners do not provide demonstrations, live or on video, that may be exploitative.

12. EH practitioners who offer educational programs take steps to ensure that graduates of their programs represent their training appropriately and with an understanding of the limitations as well as the potentials of the skills they have developed.

13. EH teachers engaged in formal supervision of EH students establish a timely and specific process for providing feedback to those they supervise, and information regarding this process is provided to the student at the beginning of supervision.

14. EH teachers do not commence sexual or romantic relationships with students in their classes and do not engage in sexual or romantic relationships with those they supervise or for whom they have evaluative responsibilities during the time they are engaged in this teaching or supervisory role.

XI. The Resolution of Ethical Issues

1. When EH practitioners believe there may have been an ethical violation by another EH practitioner, they attempt to resolve the issue by bringing it to the attention of that individual if an informal resolution appears possible and appropriate. Such interventions may not, however, violate any confidentiality rights that are involved.

2. If an apparent ethical violation has substantially harmed or is likely to substantially harm a person or organization and is not appropriate for informal resolution as described in #1, or is not adequately resolved in that fashion, EH practitioners take further action appropriate to the circumstances. Such action might include informing the appropriate ethics committee of the situation. *Exceptions:* EH practitioners are not obligated to take action based on

information gained when serving as a member of a peer review panel, as a consultant to another practitioner who is seeking consultation on the specific ethical situation in question, or as a mediator between a practitioner and one or more clients.

3.   EH practitioners do not attempt to harass, intimidate, or manipulate any person who brings a grievance before an ethics committee.

4.   EH practitioners cooperate in formal ethics investigations, proceedings, and determinations, and they submit relevant information as requested by a duly authorized ethics committee. In attempting to comply with these guidelines, they address confidentiality issues and conform to confidentiality guidelines appropriately. Failure to cooperate with an ethics investigation is itself an ethics violation.

5.   EH practitioners show respect for various personalities, rhythms, representational styles, educational levels, and backgrounds; do not falsely impugn the reputation of their colleagues; and do not file or encourage the filing of ethics complaints that are made with disregard for facts that would disprove the allegation.

6.   EH practitioners do not deny other EH practitioners employment, advancement, or admissions to training programs based solely on their being the subject of an ethics complaint. This does not preclude making decisions based on the outcome of such proceedings.

7.   EH ethics committees may take action based on information other than a formal complaint, particularly if that information is perceived by the committee as constituting a danger to the public.

8.   EH ethics committees may dismiss a claim if the client involved is unwilling to release the practitioner from confidentiality requirements that would allow a fair defense to be presented.

9.   If an EH practitioner's ethical responsibilities, as set forth in this document, conflict with a legal requirement (this may happen, for instance, if confidential health-care information is subpoenaed) or with the requirements of an organization employing the practitioner, EH practitioners make known their commitment to the ethics requirements of their professional association and take steps to resolve the conflict in a responsible manner. If the conflict is unresolvable via such means, EH practitioners may adhere to the requirements of the law or other authority according to the dictates of their conscience.

CHAPTER 5

Ethical Guidelines in a Nutshell

While reading this handbook, one of our proofreaders, Ellen Meredith, began jotting down points she wanted to remember for her own practice. Her notes comprise a useful wrap-up for the handbook, a one-page distillation, reminder, and summary, so we offer them as our closing:

- Communicate clearly with your clients about their expectations and about what you can and cannot do for them, both from the outset, and as the healing relationship evolves.

- When a questionable situation arises, inquire carefully and respectfully about your client's (or colleague's) perceptions, motivations, and stakes in the matter, and reflect on your own as well.

- Stay aware of the power dynamics in your professional settings, particularly the unequal "power" you have as a practitioner or teacher when you express opinions, offer assessments, or otherwise influence your client to think or act in a certain way.

- When faced with an unexpected ethical dilemma, identify the underlying ethical conflict and think through ways you might proceed. There is almost always a way to postpone decisive action so more information can be gathered or colleagues or other professionals consulted.

- Listen. Learn. Speak directly, clearly, and honestly to those most directly involved in an ethical situation.

- Be absolutely certain you have permission to talk about a client before doing so, and be sensitive to other confidentiality issues.

- Clean up your messes. If a situation arises in your professional activities that causes you discomfort, concern, or misgivings, bring it to your conscious attention—long before it manifests as a full-blown problem—and actively work toward resolving it.

Ethical dilemmas happen. By endeavoring to have your actions reflect the ethical principles presented in this *Ethics Handbook for Energy Healing Practitioners,* you will prevent many potential dilemmas from landing in your office, and you can navigate your way through those you do encounter more easily and gracefully. Taking the steps that prepare you to handle potential ethical dilemmas prevents them. Taking the steps to prevent potential ethical dilemmas prepares you should they occur.

Prevention is preparation. Preparation is prevention.

Appendix A

Sample Informed Consent Statements

Among the most important ways to establish an effective working relationship with your clients is to be sure they know what is being offered, what is expected of them, and what the agreements are on such key issues as confidentiality, payments, and contacting you outside scheduled appointments.

The two sample informed consent statements included here are designed for the client to read and sign prior to your first meeting. Some practitioners discuss all the relevant points in the first session or in advance on the phone, which may allow for a considerably shorter form. The versions that follow are for:

1. Certified Eden Energy Medicine practitioners
2. Energy psychology practitioners who are licensed mental health–care providers

For Reiki, Healing Touch, non-licensed EFT practitioners, and the wide variety of other energy healers, very little wording needs to be changed on one or the other of the following forms. To make this easier, electronic versions of these forms that can be customized are available in the *Toolkit for Energy Healing Practitioners,* a program available for PC and Mac computers, which includes more than seventy-five documents relevant for developing an energy healing practice.

Sample informed consent statements for energy healing practitioners, EFT practitioners, or other energy psychology practitioners who prefer to operate as life coaches (energy enhancement coaches or peak performance coaches) are also available in the *Toolkit.*

For further information about the *Toolkit,* visit *http://toolkit.inner-source.net.*

Sample Informed Consent for
Energy Medicine Practitioners

Introduction

Obtaining informed consent is one of the most fundamental procedures for protecting a client's rights. Informed consent means that prior to establishing a professional relationship, the prospective client has been provided with enough information to make a reasonable determination about whether to enlist the services you offer. This information includes the goals of your services, the procedures, and your qualifications; warnings about possible side effects; information about fees, length and frequency of sessions, and the likely duration of the professional relationship; and alternative services that might be sought for reaching the same goals. The differences between your services and the services provided by a licensed health-care professional should be made particularly explicit. Essential for informed consent is that the client be able to understand this information and be able to choose freely whether to proceed with the services. Having the client sign a statement early in (or prior to) the first session is one of the most basic ways that informed consent can be responsibly obtained.

The following informed consent statement can be used as a rough model as you develop your own. State laws differ in what may be practiced without a license and the language that may be used. Your informed consent statement may be your first formal communication with your client, so you will want to personalize it as appropriate and be sure it is consistent with pertinent laws and regulations. In addition to providing information that helps the client understand your services, the following sample aims to establish a legally enforceable business relationship with the client. Doing this well minimizes the risk of the misunderstandings that could become the basis for ethical complaints or malpractice suits. This form uses the language for Eden Energy Medicine Certified Practitioners, but can easily be adapted for Reiki, Healing Touch, or other certified energy healing professionals. A separate form for life energy coaches can be found in the *Toolkit for Energy Healing Practitioners (http://toolkit.innersource.net)*.

The following includes some general language about risks and benefits, but because these can vary considerably, the risk and benefits should be supplemented orally or in writing by the practitioners. No single document is appropriate for all situations. For example, it is probably important to have a more thorough discussion of risks and benefits with clients who are seeking your help and who also have a serious medical condition. The goal is to have no misunderstandings about the limitations or the scope of the services you offer. Steps that should be followed if the condition worsens can then be considered.

An informed consent agreement is only the beginning of providing informed consent. Important issues contained in the agreement, or not contained in it, should be discussed when it is anticipated that such issues are likely to occur. This is particularly important if the client is likely to feel betrayed or feel angry should these issues arise, as in instances in which you are required to disclose confidential information. You may orally provide whatever additional information is necessary and make a note in the client's record about what was said.

Laws relating to client access to personal records, confidentiality, and testimonial privilege differ from state to state and profession to profession. In the spirit of informed consent, you are strongly advised to have an attorney who knows the specific laws in your state and your specialty review a draft of the consent form you plan to use. Also take care that your final version does not include language that could be interpreted as a guarantee or implied warranty regarding the services rendered.

Feel free to adapt the following draft for your practice or setting. It builds on an earlier sample informed consent statement for energy practitioners provided by Douglas J. Moore, PhD, as well as two other informed consent statements graciously provided by Laura S. Brown, PhD, ABPP, and by Bruce E. Bennett, PhD, and Eric Harris, JD, EdD.

DISCLAIMER: This document is not necessarily appropriate in all aspects for your situation nor is it a substitute for legal consultation.

[YOUR LETTERHEAD]

Energy Medicine Services Disclosure Statement And Agreement

Welcome! This document contains important information about my professional services and business policies. It is rather long because it covers a wide range of possible situations, many of which will not apply to you. Still, it provides a framework for understanding the services you are considering. Please read it carefully and note any questions you might have. We can discuss them at our next meeting. If you decide to use my services and sign this document, it will represent an agreement between us.

What Is Energy Medicine?

I am a certified practitioner of Eden Energy Medicine. Energy medicine is an approach that involves balancing and restoring your body's natural energies for the purposes of increasing your vitality, strengthening your mental capacities, and optimizing your health. The form I use draws from Donna Eden and her book *Energy Medicine*.

Roots. The techniques you will be experiencing and learning trace back to ancient healing and spiritual traditions such as yoga, tai chi, and acupuncture. The variety I use and teach is thoroughly modern and does not require adherence to any particular set of beliefs or practices. The core concept is that your personal well-being and effectiveness are directly related to the state of your body's energies.

Your Body's Energies. Einstein's famous formula, $E = mc^2$, changed the course of physics and of history by showing that matter is a form of energy. Our bodies are comprised of molecules that are in constant motion and that are continually being influenced by outside forces. The medical profession measures electromagnetic fields with devices such as EKGs, EEGs, and MRIs. The vital role these energies play in our everyday health and well-being is well established. Scientists from a range of disciplines are now introducing concepts such as "force fields" and "subtle energies" to explain a range of empirical observations. Subtle energies are called "subtle" because they are not easily detectable and scientists have not been able to develop instruments to measure them reliably. Nonetheless, people throughout history and across cultures have described seeing or feeling subtle energies.

Enhancing Your Body's Energies. You may have heard about subtle energy through terms such as the "life force," "chi," "meridians," "chakras," "biofields," or "auras." In many healing traditions, the "life force," the animating power whose presence defines life and whose absence defines death, is understood as a form of subtle energy. Eastern cultures, in particular, have studied such energies for millennia and have successfully applied their understanding for enhancing both physical and emotional health. Systems designed to influence the body's subtle energies include yoga, Reiki, acupuncture, acupressure, tai chi, therapeutic touch, and energy medicine, to name just a few. Many hospitals in the United States now include such methods to help with the healing of a variety of conditions.

Energy Medicine Techniques. The techniques I will be using and teaching you are based on the premise that by promoting balance and flow in the body's electromagnetic and subtle energies, health and well-being are enhanced. The techniques may involve the use of certain postures or movements or touching, holding, pressing on, tracing, or circling over specified areas of the skin. They move, balance, enhance, and restore the body's energies. I may also employ a procedure called "energy testing" where I apply light pressure to your outstretched arm, sometimes while you or I touch another area of your body. This is a way of assessing how your energies are flowing through specific areas of your body and may help us identify the techniques that will be most beneficial for you. The methods we will be using lend themselves to highly individualized applications in the office as well as to back-home self-care.

What Are the Limitations of My Energy Medicine Practice?

Although energy medicine uses the term "medicine," it does not imply that energy medicine practitioners are practicing medicine. Energy medicine is a term used by many training programs that teach people how to assess and correct for energy imbalances in the body. Energy medicine is not a substitute for the diagnosis and/or treatment of medical or mental health conditions by a licensed health-care professional. If you have a disorder that has been diagnosed by a licensed medical or mental health professional or a condition that should be evaluated by a licensed health professional, my services should be used only in conjunction with your obtaining that care. I do not diagnose or treat medical or mental health disorders, nor am I trained or licensed to do so. Energy medicine attempts to optimize the body's overall health and vitality, but it is not to be used instead of appropriate care from a licensed professional.

Besides the fact that energy medicine does not diagnose or treat illness, another difference between my services and typical visits to a medical doctor is that effective energy work requires your active involvement between sessions. Our sessions will establish energy patterns that optimize body, mind, and spirit. Reinforcing these new patterns through the practice of energy exercises at home will reinforce, maintain, and extend the benefits you receive in the sessions.

Energy medicine techniques bring disturbed energies back to a state of balance and harmony. These corrections will generally consist of various forms of light or deeper touch and of movement of my hands within your body's energy field. If you are uncomfortable with being touched or with any of the procedures being used, please tell me immediately and I will instantly stop.

While the methods I use and teach are gentle and considered non-invasive, it is possible that physical or emotional aftereffects may occur after your energies have been stimulated and adjusted. In some instances, deeper pressure is used to move energies that may be blocked or congested in a particular area of the body, and this may cause some pain or discomfort. Dizziness, nausea, and anxiety are relatively unusual but not unheard of side effects to energy work. If any procedure is disquieting or leads to discomfort, please tell me at once. I will instantly stop if you request me to do so and can often provide a technique to counter the discomfort.

My Background and Training

[Include degrees, certificates, licenses, institutions, specialties, philosophy, etc.]

Meetings

I generally schedule one appointment of ninety-minutes' duration per week, at a time we agree upon. Sessions may also, by prior agreement, be longer, shorter, more frequent, or less frequent.

Professional Records

I keep brief records on each session, primarily noting the date of the session, the interventions used, and progress or obstacles observed as they relate to your goals in working with me. You are welcome to request, in writing, that I make available to other health-care providers a copy of your file. I maintain your records in a secure location that cannot be accessed by anyone else. I will maintain your records for at least seven years after our last contact, after which time I may securely dispose of them.

Confidentiality

[Some provisions will vary on a state-by-state basis.]

With the exception of special situations described in the numbered list that follows, you have the absolute right to the confidentiality of your therapy. I cannot and will not tell anyone else what you have told me, or even that you are in therapy with me without your prior written permission. Under the provisions of the Health Care Information Act of 1992, I may under certain circumstances legally speak to another health-care provider or a member of your family about you without your prior consent, but I will not do so unless the situation is an emergency. I will always act so as to protect your privacy to the best of my ability. You may direct me to share information with whomever you choose, and you can change your mind and revoke that permission at any time. You may request anyone you wish to attend a session with you.

You are also protected under the provisions of the Federal Health Insurance Portability and Accountability Act (HIPAA). This law ensures the confidentiality of all electronic transmission of information about you. Whenever I transmit information about you electronically (for example, sending bills to your insurance company), it will be done with special safeguards such as a secure server to ensure confidentiality. If you elect to communicate with me by e-mail at some point in our work together, please be aware that e-mail is not completely confidential. All e-mails are retained in the logs of your or my Internet service provider. Although under normal circumstances no one looks at these logs, they are, in theory, available to be read by the system administrators of the Internet service provider. As part of your treatment record, I will keep any e-mail I receive from you, and any responses that I send to you.

Following are seven exceptions to your right to confidentiality:

1. There are some situations in which I am legally obligated to take action to protect others from harm, even if I have to reveal some information about a client's treatment. For example, if I believe that a child, an elderly person, or a disabled person is being abused, I must file a report with the appropriate state or local agency.

2. If I believe that a client is threatening serious bodily harm to another, I am required to take protective actions. These actions may include notifying the potential victim, contacting the police, or seeking hospitalization for the client.

3. If I believe that you are in imminent danger of harming yourself, I may legally break confidentiality and contact the police, a local crisis team, or a family member or other intimates.

4. If you tell me of the behavior of another named health or mental health–care provider that suggests this person has either (1) engaged in sexual contact with a patient, including yourself, or (2) is impaired from practice in some manner due to cognitive, emotional, behavioral, or health problems, then the law requires me [this particularly varies by state] to report this to the practitioner's state licensing board. I would inform you before taking this step. If you are my client and are also a health-care provider, however, your confidentiality remains protected under the law from this kind of reporting.

5. In certain legal proceedings, particularly those involving child custody or those in which your emotional condition or treatment is an important issue, a judge may order my testimony. Confidentiality is not protected when a judge makes such an order or in certain other legal procedures. Consult with an attorney if you are involved in a legal situation in which such confidentialities may be at issue.

6. If am asked to provide services to your spouse, partner, or another member of your family, we will in advance establish the limits of confidentiality. It generally confines a practitioner's effectiveness when required to keep secrets, so my policy in most circumstances is that what you say and what we do *can* be shared with other family members I am working with. If this is what we establish, *do not tell me anything you wish kept secret* from other intimates who are receiving sessions from me. If confidential information is a concern, it may be better for each family member to work with a different practitioner.

7. I may occasionally find it helpful to consult other professionals about a client. During a consultation, I make every effort to avoid revealing the identity of the client. The consultant is also bound to keep the information confidential. If you don't object, I will not tell you about these consultations unless I feel that it is important to our work together.

Although this written summary of exceptions to confidentiality should prove helpful in informing you about potential problems, please discuss with me any questions or concerns you may have. I will be happy to explore these issues with you, but formal legal advice may be needed from an attorney because the laws governing confidentiality can be quite complex.

Minors

If you are under eighteen years of age, please be aware that the law may provide your parents or legal guardians the right to examine my records of our work together. It is my policy to request a written agreement from parents to waive their right to access your records. If they agree, I will provide them only with general information about our work together unless I feel there is a high risk that you will seriously harm yourself or someone else. In this case, I will notify them of my concern. Before giving them any information, I will discuss the matter with you, if possible, and do my best to handle any objections you may have about what I am planning to discuss.

[The laws on providing health-care services to minors without parental consent vary from state to state—be sure your wording is consistent with the local regulations.]

Professional Fees

My fee for a ninety-minute session is [$XXX]. If we decide to meet for a longer session or a shorter session, I will bill you prorated on this hourly fee. In addition to scheduled appointments, I also prorate the hourly fee for other professional services you may request. Other services might include emergency telephone conversations lasting longer than ten minutes, listening to lengthy voice mail messages, reading and responding to e-mails other than for routine business, attending meetings with other professionals you have authorized, and preparing requested records or treatment summaries. If you become involved in legal proceedings that require my participation, you will be expected to pay for my professional time even if I am called to testify by another party. Because of the difficulty of legal involvement, I charge [$XXX] per hour for preparation and attendance at any legal proceeding.

Billing and Payments

You will be expected to pay for each session at the time it is held unless we agree otherwise. Payment schedules for other professional services will be agreed to when they are requested.

Once an appointment is scheduled, you will be expected to pay for it unless you provide twenty-four-hours' advance notice of cancellation. If you are late, we will still end on time and not run over into the next person's session. If you miss a session without canceling, or cancel with less than twenty-four-hours' notice, you must pay for that session by the time of our next meeting unless we both agree that you were unable to attend due to circumstances beyond your control. In circumstances of unusual financial hardship, I may be willing to negotiate a payment installment plan.

If that is done and your account has not been paid for more than sixty days and arrangements for payment have not been agreed upon, I have the option of using legal means to secure the payment. This may involve hiring a collection agency or going through small claims court. If such legal action is necessary, its costs will be included in the claim. In most collection situations, the only information released is the client's name, contact information, dates and type of services provided, and the amount due.

Contacting Me

I am often with a client or otherwise not immediately available by telephone. When I am unavailable, you will reach my voice mail. I monitor it frequently and will make every effort to return your call on the same day you make it, with the exception of weekends and holidays. If it will be difficult to reach you, please inform me of some times when you will be available. If you are unable to reach me and feel that you can't wait for me to return your call, contact your family physician or, if you are experiencing a medical emergency, call 911 or go to the emergency room of a nearby hospital.

Other Aspects of Our Relationship

You have the right to ask me questions about anything that happens in our work together. I'm always willing to discuss how and why I've decided to do what I'm doing, and to look at alternatives that might work better. You can feel free to ask me to try something that you think will be helpful. You can ask me about my training for working with your concerns and can request that I refer you to someone else if you decide I'm not the right practitioner for you. You are free to terminate our work together at any time.

I never engage in sexual intimacies with clients or former clients and generally avoid social and business relationships. Beyond the legal and ethical considerations, our work together will be most effective when kept free from possible outside entanglements.

Touch. Physical contact, even in a healing relationship, can be a sensitive matter because touch can be easily misinterpreted and feel too intimate, uncomfortable, or sexual in nature. Touching in a sexual manner is unethical within a professional healing relationship, illegal, and will never be a part of your treatment. Many of the methods I will use, however, are likely to involve touch. The theory behind such methods is that touching or holding points can assist me, and you, in identifying and shifting imbalances in your energies. At such times, you would remain fully clothed, with perhaps the exception of your shoes. I will always explain ahead of time where I will touch, and you can let me know if you are comfortable with it or not. I will always honor any requests not to touch.

Touch can also be a potential problem in a healing relationship if you have had a history of paranoia, have been diagnosed with borderline personality disorder, have been sexually or physically abused, have suffered from other types of trauma, or if you tend to dissociate or detach from your sense of self. Prior to our starting our work together, please let me know if you fall into any of these categories. We can discuss any emotional risks associated with touch that may be of concern to you. Furthermore, if you have any misgivings, doubts, or any negative reactions to any physical contact, it is very important that you let me know as soon as possible so that we can discuss your concerns. If you are uncomfortable talking to me, I encourage you to talk through such concerns with another professional. If you wish, I can make a referral for you.

Legal Proceedings. If you are involved in legal proceedings based on your having been traumatized, please understand that the goals of our work together may involve healing the physical and emotional aftermath of the trauma, and this could adversely affect your ability to provide legal testimony that carries the same impact as it would prior to treatment.

Terminating Treatment. Normally, you will be the one who decides when our work together will end, but there are three exceptions to this. If I determine that I am unable, for any reason, to provide you with the services you are requesting at a high professional standard, I will inform you of this decision and refer you to another practitioner who may better meet your needs. Second, if you verbally or physically threaten or harass me, my office, or my family, I reserve the right to terminate you from treatment immediately and unilaterally. Third, I reserve the right to refuse or terminate a session if you or anyone in the session is suspected of being under the influence of a mood-altering substance. You will be responsible and charged for full payment of the normal fee.

Vacations. I am away from the office several times each year for vacations or to attend professional meetings. I will make every effort to tell you well in advance of any anticipated lengthy absences and to discuss other options for continuing to work toward your goals during my absence.

Complaints

If you are unhappy with the way our work together is proceeding, I hope you will talk about it with me so that I can respond directly to your concerns. I will take such concerns seriously and meet them with care and respect. You are also free to discuss any complaints about me with anyone you wish. You do not have any responsibility to maintain confidentiality about what I say or do. You are the person who has the right to decide what you want kept confidential. If you believe that I have been unwilling to listen and respond, or that I have behaved unethically, you can register a complaint about my behavior with the organization that certifies me as an Eden Energy Medicine practitioner:

Innersource
777 East Main Street
Ashland, OR 97520
541-482-1800
www.innersource.net ethics@innersource.org.

Your signature below indicates that you have read the information in this document, understand it fully, have discussed any questions or matters of concern with me and/or others, and agree to abide by its terms during our professional relationship.

_____   _____
            Print Name   Date

_____
            Signature

Sample Informed Consent Statement for Psychotherapists Using Energy Psychology

Introduction

Obtaining informed consent is one of the most fundamental procedures for protecting a client's rights. Informed consent means that prior to establishing a therapeutic relationship, the prospective client has been provided with enough information to make a reasonable determination about whether to enlist the services you offer. This information includes the procedures and goals of the psychotherapy; the qualifications of and approach used by the therapist; warnings about possible side effects; information about fees, length and frequency of sessions, and likely duration of treatment; alternative therapeutic approaches; and potential sources of help besides psychotherapy. Essential for informed consent is that the client be able to understand this information and be able to choose freely whether to proceed with the treatment. Having the client sign a statement early in (or prior to) the treatment is one of the most basic ways that informed consent can be responsibly obtained.

The following informed consent statement can be used as a rough model as you develop your own. Because state laws and individual licensing boards differ in what they require, and your informed consent statement may be your first formal communication with your client, you will want to personalize it as appropriate and be sure it is consistent with pertinent laws and regulations. The following sample, in addition to providing information that helps the client understand your services, aims to establish a legally enforceable business relationship with the client. Doing this well minimizes the risk of the misunderstandings that could become the basis for ethical complaints or malpractice suits.

This draft was designed for psychotherapy practices. It can and should be modified to include other practice areas such as allied health care, neuropsychological assessments, family therapy, or group psychotherapy. A paragraph that introduces energy psychology is included.

The draft includes some general language about the risks and benefits of psychotherapy, but because it may vary considerably, the risks and benefits should be supplemented orally or in writing by the therapist on a case-by-case basis. No single document is appropriate for all situations. For example, it is probably important to have a more thorough discussion of risks and benefits with clients who are at high risk of self-harm or who are in an abusive relationship. You can orally provide whatever additional information is necessary and make a note in the client's record about what was said. Of course, this will not be as protective as a signed agreement, but in most cases it makes both clinical and risk management sense.

An informed consent agreement is only the beginning of providing informed consent. Important issues contained in the agreement, or not contained in it, should be discussed when it is anticipated that they are likely to occur. This is particularly important if the client is likely to feel betrayed or feel angry should these issues arise, as in instances in which you are required to disclose confidential information.

Laws relating to client access to personal records, confidentiality, and testimonial privilege differ from state to state and profession to profession. In the spirit of informed consent, you are strongly advised to have an attorney who knows the specific laws in your state and for your specialty review a draft of the consent form you plan to use. Also take care that your final version does not include language that could be interpreted as a guarantee or implied warranty regarding the services rendered.

Feel free to adapt the following draft for your practice or setting. It builds on an earlier sample informed consent statement for energy practitioners provided by Douglas J. Moore, PhD, as well as two other informed consent statements graciously provided by Laura S. Brown, PhD, ABPP, and by Bruce E. Bennett, PhD, and Eric Harris, JD, EdD.

DISCLAIMER: This document is not necessarily appropriate in all aspects for your situation nor is it a substitute for legal consultation.

[YOUR LETTERHEAD]

Psychotherapy Disclosure Statement and Agreement

Welcome! This document contains important information about my professional services and business policies. It is rather long because it covers a wide range of possible situations, many of which will not apply to you. Still, it provides a framework for understanding the services you are considering. Please read it carefully and note any questions you might have. We can discuss them at our next meeting. If you decide to use my services and sign this document, it will represent an agreement between us.

Psychological Services

Psychotherapy is not easily described in general statements. It varies depending on the training of the psychologist, the personalities of both the psychologist and client, and the particular problems the client brings forward. There are many different methods I may use to deal with the problems that you hope to address. Psychotherapy calls for a very active effort on your part. For the therapy to be most successful, it will be in your best interest to work on things we talk about both during our sessions and at home.

Psychotherapy can have risks as well as benefits. Since therapy often involves discussing unpleasant aspects of your life, you may experience uncomfortable feelings like sadness, guilt, anger, frustration, loneliness, and helplessness. Making changes in your beliefs or behaviors can be unsettling and sometimes disruptive to the relationships you already have. You may find your relationship with me to be a source of strong feelings, some of them unpleasant at times. It is important that you consider carefully whether these risks are worth the potential benefits to you of attaining your goals in seeking help. Most people who take these risks find that therapy is helpful. Therapy often leads to better relationships, solutions to specific problems, and significant reductions in feelings of distress. But there are no guarantees of what you will experience.

The early part of our work together will involve an evaluation of your needs. By the end of the evaluation, I will be able to offer you some first impressions of what our work might include and an initial approach if you decide to continue with therapy. You should evaluate this information in light of your own opinions and whether you feel comfortable working with me. Therapy involves the commitment of time, money, and energy, so you should be very careful about the therapist you select. If you have questions about my procedures, we should discuss them whenever they arise. If your doubts persist, I will be happy to help you set up a meeting with another mental health professional for a second opinion.

My Background and Training

[Include degrees, certificates, licenses, institutions, specialties, philosophy, etc.]

My Approach to Psychotherapy

Our work together is likely to include some or all of the following: dialogue, goal-setting, problem-solving, investigation of how your current concerns may have their roots in your earlier experiences, examination of our therapeutic relationship as a prototype of other relationships in your life, stress-reduction techniques, exploration of unconscious motivation, and a review of your experiences since the last session as they pertain to your therapeutic goals. [Adjust as appropriate.] I may suggest that you consult with a medical professional or other specialist to work in conjunction with the services I provide. If another specialist is working with you, I will most likely need a release of information from you so that I can communicate freely with that person about your care. You have the right to refuse anything that I suggest.

Energy Psychology. In addition to the more conventional methods listed previously, I utilize an approach known as energy psychology. The roots of energy psychology trace back to Eastern healing practices that work with the acupuncture points, the chakras, and the body's energy systems. The method usually involves having you tap with your fingers on specific areas of the skin while bringing to mind a personal response or pattern you would like to change. This is believed to shift the brain's chemistry in ways that support that change. Other verbalizations and physical movements may also be used. I may also employ a procedure called "energy testing," in which I apply light pressure to your out-stretched arm while you make a statement based on wording that I suggest. This is a way of assessing how certain thoughts you have may lead to disruptions in your body's energies as well as being a way of assessing progress. Energy psychology is still considered an "experimental treatment," although early research has been promising. A professional paper that reviews this research and speculates on why the method seems to work can be downloaded free from *www.EnergyPsychEd.com/mechanisms*. I have received professional training in the use of these techniques and will be happy to discuss them with you. If you prefer not to use these techniques or to discontinue their use at any point, that is entirely your call.

Meetings

I generally schedule one appointment of fifty-minutes' duration per week, at a time we agree upon. Sessions may also, by prior agreement, be longer, shorter, more frequent, or less frequent.

Professional Records

I keep brief records on each session, primarily noting the date of the session, the topics discussed, the interventions used, and progress or obstacles observed as they relate to your treatment goals. Under the provisions of the Health Care Information Act of 1992, you have the right to a copy of your file at any time. You have the right to request that I correct any errors in your file. You have the right, at your written request, to have me make available to any other health-care provider a copy of your file. I maintain your records in a secure location that cannot be accessed by anyone else.

I will maintain your records for at least seven years after our last contact, after which time I may securely dispose of them.

Confidentiality

[Some provisions will vary on a state-by-state basis.]

With the exception of special situations described in the numbered list that follows, you have the absolute right to the confidentiality of your therapy. I cannot and will not tell anyone else what you have told me, or even that you are in therapy with me, without your prior written permission. Under the provisions of the Health Care Information Act of 1992, I may under certain circumstances legally speak to another health-care provider or a member of your family about you without your prior consent, but I will not do so unless the situation is an emergency. I will always act so as to protect your privacy to the best of my ability. You may direct me to share information with whomever you chose, and you can change your mind and revoke that permission at any time. You may request anyone you wish to attend a therapy session with you.

You are also protected under the provisions of the Federal Health Insurance Portability and Accountability Act (HIPAA). This law ensures the confidentiality of all electronic transmission of information about you. Whenever I transmit information about you electronically (for example, sending bills to your insurance company), it will be done with special safeguards such as a secure server to ensure confidentiality. If you elect to communicate with me by e-mail at some point in our work together, please be aware that e-mail is not completely confidential. All e-mails are retained in the logs of your or my Internet service provider. Although under normal circumstances no one looks at these logs, they are, in theory, available to be read by the system administrators of the Internet service provider. As part of your treatment record, I will keep any e-mail I receive from you, and any responses that I send to you.

Following are seven exceptions to your right to confidentiality:

1. There are some situations in which I am legally obligated to take action to protect others from harm, even if I have to reveal some information about a client's treatment. For example, if I believe that a child, an

elderly person, or a disabled person is being abused, I must file a report with the appropriate state or local agency.

2. If I believe that a client is threatening serious bodily harm to another, I am required to take protective actions. These actions may include notifying the potential victim, contacting the police, or seeking hospitalization for the client.

3. If I believe that you are in imminent danger of harming yourself, I may legally break confidentiality and contact the police, a local crisis team, or a family member or other intimates.

4. If you tell me of the behavior of another named health or mental health–care provider that suggests this person has either (1) engaged in sexual contact with a patient, including yourself, or (2) is impaired from practice in some manner due to cognitive, emotional, behavioral, or health problems, then the law requires me [this particularly varies by state] to report this to the practitioner's state licensing board. I would inform you before taking this step. If you are my client and also a health-care provider, however, your confidentiality remains protected under the law from this kind of reporting.

5. In certain legal proceedings, particularly those involving child custody or those in which your emotional condition or treatment is an important issue, a judge may order my testimony. Confidentiality is not protected when a judge makes such an order or in certain other legal procedures. Consult with an attorney if you are involved in a legal situation in which such confidentialities may be at issue.

6. The following is not a legal exception to your confidentiality, but it is a policy you should be aware of if you are in couples therapy or family therapy with me. If you and your partner or other adult family member decide to have some individual sessions as part of the couples or family therapy, what you say in those individual sessions will be considered to be a part of the couples or family therapy. It can and very possibly will be discussed in our joint sessions. Do not tell me anything you wish kept secret from the others involved in the therapy.

7. I may occasionally find it helpful to consult other professionals about a case. During a consultation, I make every effort to avoid revealing the identity of my client. The consultant is also legally bound to keep the

information confidential. If you don't object, I will not tell you about these consultations unless I feel that it is important to our work together.

Although this written summary of exceptions to confidentiality should prove helpful in informing you about potential problems, please discuss with me any questions or concerns you may have. I will be happy to explore these issues with you, but formal legal advice may be needed from an attorney because the laws governing confidentiality can be quite complex.

Minors

If you are under eighteen years of age, please be aware that the law may provide your parents or legal guardians the right to examine your treatment records. It is my policy to request a written agreement from parents to waive their right to access your records. If they agree, I will provide them only with general information about our work together unless I feel there is a high risk that you will seriously harm yourself or someone else. In this case, I will notify them of my concern. I will also provide them with a general summary of your treatment when it is complete. Before giving them any information, I will discuss the matter with you, if possible, and do my best to handle any objections you may have about what I am planning to discuss.

[The laws on providing health-care services to minors without parental consent vary from state to state—be sure your wording is consistent with the local regulations.]

Professional Fees

My hourly fee is [$XXX] (includes the fifty-minute session and related routine record keeping). If we decide to meet for a longer session or a shorter session, I will bill you prorated on this hourly fee. In addition to scheduled appointments, I also prorate the hourly fee for other professional services you may request. Other services might include emergency telephone conversations lasting longer than ten minutes, listening to lengthy voice mail messages, reading and responding to e-mails other than for routine business, attending meetings with other professionals you have authorized, and preparing requested records or treatment summaries. If you become involved in legal proceedings that require my participation, you will be expected to pay for my professional time even if I am called to testify by another party. Because of the difficulty of legal involvement, I charge [$XXX] per hour for preparation and attendance at any legal proceeding.

Billing and Payments

You will be expected to pay for each session at the time it is held unless we agree otherwise or unless you have insurance coverage that requires another arrangement. Payment schedules for other professional services will be agreed to when they are requested.

Once an appointment is scheduled, you will be expected to pay for it unless you provide twenty-four-hours' advance notice of cancellation. If you are late, we will still end on time and not run over into the next person's session. If you miss a session without canceling, or cancel with less than twenty-four–hours' notice, you must pay for that session by the time of our next meeting unless we both agree that you were unable to attend due to circumstances beyond your control. In circumstances of unusual financial hardship, I may be willing to negotiate a payment installment plan.

If that is done and your account has not been paid for more than sixty days and arrangements for payment have not been agreed upon, I have the option of using legal means to secure the payment. This may involve hiring a collection agency or going through small claims court. If such legal action is necessary, its costs will be included in the claim. In most collection situations, the only information released regarding a client's treatment is name, contact information, dates and type of services provided, and the amount due.

Insurance Reimbursement

In order for us to set realistic treatment goals and priorities, it is important to evaluate what resources you have available to pay for your treatment. If you have a health insurance policy, it will usually provide some coverage for mental health treatment. I will fill out forms and provide you with whatever assistance I can in helping you receive the benefits to which you are entitled; however, you (not your insurance company) are responsible for full payment of my fees. It is very important that you find out exactly what mental health services your insurance policy covers.

You should carefully read the section in your insurance coverage booklet that describes mental health services. If you have questions about the coverage, call your plan administrator. Of course, I will provide you with whatever information I can based on my experience and will be happy to help you in understanding the information you receive from your insurance company. If it is necessary to clear confusion, I will be willing to call the company on your behalf.

Due to the rising costs of health care, insurance benefits have become more complex. It is sometimes difficult to determine exactly how much mental health coverage is available. "Managed care" plans such as HMOs and PPOs often require authorization before they provide reimbursement for mental health services. These plans are often limited to short-term treatment approaches designed to work out specific problems that interfere with a person's usual level of functioning. It may be necessary to seek approval for more therapy after a certain number of sessions. Although a lot can be accomplished in short-term therapy, some clients feel that they need more services after insurance benefits end. In rare cases, an insurance plan will not allow the same therapist to provide services once benefits end. If this is the case, I will do my best to find another provider who will help you continue your psychotherapy.

You should also be aware that most insurance companies require you to authorize me to provide them with a clinical diagnosis. Sometimes I have to provide additional clinical information such as treatment plans or summaries, or copies of the entire record. This information will become part of the insurance company files and will probably be stored in a computer. Though all insurance companies claim to keep such information confidential, I have no control over what they do with it once it is in their hands. In some cases, they may share some of this information with a national medical information databank. I will provide you with a copy of any report I submit, if you request it.

Once we have all of the information about your insurance coverage, we will discuss what we can expect to accomplish with the benefits that are available and what will happen if they run out before you feel ready to end our sessions. It is important to remember that you always have the right to pay for my services yourself to avoid the problems and complications described here.

Contacting Me

I am often with a client or otherwise not immediately available by telephone. When I am unavailable, my telephone is answered by my secretary or by voice mail. I monitor my voice mail frequently and will make every effort to return your call on the same day you make it, with the exception of weekends and holidays. If it will be difficult to reach you, please inform me of some times when you will be available. If you are unable to reach me and feel that you can't wait for me to return your call, contact your family physician or the [[Name] Crisis Clinic at XXX-XXX-XXXX]. If you believe that you cannot keep yourself safe, please call 911 or go to the emergency room of a nearby hospital and ask for the psychiatrist or psychologist on call. If I will be unavailable for an extended time, I will provide you with the name of a colleague to contact if necessary.

Other Aspects of Our Relationship

I Welcome Your Questions. You have the right to ask me questions about anything that happens in our work together. I'm always willing to discuss how and why I've decided to do what I'm doing, and to look at alternatives that might work better. You can feel free to ask me to try something that you think will be helpful. You can ask me about my training for working with your concerns and can request that I refer you to someone else if you decide I'm not the right practitioner for you. You are free to terminate our work together at any time.

    Contacts Outside Our Work Together. I generally avoid social and business relationships with my clients. Our work together will be most effective when kept free from possible outside entanglements. I, of course, never engage in sexual intimacies with clients.

    Psychotherapeutic Touch. Physical contact within psychotherapy has sometimes been frowned upon because touch can be easily misinterpreted and feel too intimate, uncomfortable, or sexual in nature. Touching in a sexual manner is unethical within psychotherapy, illegal, and will never be a part of your treatment. There are times, however, when it is beneficial for me to hold certain points on your body. The theory behind such methods is that touching or holding these points can assist me, and you, in identifying and shifting imbalances in your energies. If there are such times, you would remain fully clothed, with perhaps the exception of your shoes. I will always explain ahead of time where I will touch, and you can let me know if you are comfortable with it or not. I will always honor any requests not to touch.

Touch can also be a potential problem in a therapeutic relationship if you have had a history of paranoia, have been diagnosed with borderline personality disorder, have been sexually or physically abused, have suffered from other types of trauma, or if you tend to dissociate or detach from your sense of self. Prior to our starting our work together, please let me know if you fall into any of these categories. We can discuss any emotional risks associated with touch that may be of concern to you. Furthermore, if you have any misgivings, doubts, or any negative reactions to any physical contact, it is very important that you let me know as soon as possible so that we can discuss your concerns. If you are uncomfortable talking to me, I encourage you to talk through such concerns with another professional. If you wish, I can make a referral for you.

Legal Proceedings. If you are involved in legal proceedings based on your having been traumatized, please understand that the goals of our work together may involve healing the physical and emotional aftermath of the trauma, and this could adversely affect your ability to provide legal testimony that carries the same impact as it would prior to treatment.

Terminating Treatment. Normally, you will be the one who decides when therapy will end, but there are three exceptions to this. If I determine that I am unable, for any reason, to provide you with the services you are requesting at a high professional standard, I will inform you of this decision and refer you to another therapist who may better meet your needs. Second, if you verbally or physically threaten or harass me, my office, or my family, I reserve the right to terminate you from treatment immediately and unilaterally. Third, I reserve the right to refuse or terminate a session if you or anyone in the session is suspected of being under the influence of a mood-altering substance. You will be responsible and charged for full payment of the normal fee.

Vacations. I am away from the office several times each year for vacations or to attend professional meetings. If I am not receiving or responding to phone or e-mail messages during those times, I will have someone cover my practice. I will tell you well in advance of any anticipated lengthy absences and give you the name and phone number of the therapist who will be covering my practice during my absence.

Complaints

If you are unhappy with the way your therapy is proceeding, I hope you will talk about it with me so that I can respond directly to your concerns. I will take such concerns seriously and meet them with care and respect. You are also free to discuss any complaints about me with anyone you wish. You do not have any responsibility to maintain confidentiality about what I say or do. You are the person who has the right to decide what you want kept confidential. If you believe that I have been unwilling to listen and respond, or that I have behaved unethically, you can register a complaint about my behavior with the State Board of [include exact name, address, phone, and website as appropriate].

Your signature below indicates that you have read the information in this document, understand it fully, have discussed any questions or matters of concern with me and/or others, and agree to abide by its terms during our professional relationship.

_____   _____

Print Name   Date

_____

Signature

Sample Instructions for Submitting Ethics Complaints

Following is the actual document used by for ethics complaints pertaining to Eden Energy Medicine (EEM) Certified Practitioners. It is provided here for our sister organizations to consider in developing their own procedures for receiving ethical complaints and to inform readers of the *Ethics Handbook for Energy Healing Practitioners* about how ethical complaints may be submitted within a professional organization.

Instructions for Submitting an Ethics Complaint

This document provides instruction for the significant action of formally submitting an ethics complaint about an Eden Energy Medicine (EEM) practitioner, student, teaching assistant (TA), or faculty member.

A challenge for any ethics review process is that the responsibility of stopping unethical or harmful behavior on the part of a practitioner must be balanced with the responsibility of seeing that a practitioner is not condemned based on hearsay or other insufficient evidence. The EEM Ethics Committee Overview and Procedures (see appendix 3) attempt to ensure that both concerns are met. Specific points to keep in mind include:

1. The first step after learning of a possible ethics violation by a colleague, as described in the *Ethics Handbook for Energy Healing Practitioners*, is to try within reasonable limits to resolve the ethics issues directly with that person. If you are not persuaded that this can be or has been accomplished, an ethics complaint may be appropriate.

2. Before submitting an ethics complaint, please be sure that you are proceeding with reasonable certainty in bringing the charges. It is not unknown for the person submitting a complaint to subsequently be the subject of an ethics complaint or a lawsuit brought by the individual about whom the complaint was registered. Be sure that your formal complaint is not vulnerable to charges of being frivolous or unfounded. To help orient you to the issues you should consider, guidelines taken from the "Ethics Code for Energy Healing Practitioners" are summarized at the end of this document. If you are unsure of your responsibilities or the grounds for your complaint, consider consulting with a colleague or an attorney.

3. As with many professional ethics complaint procedures, Innersource, the organization overseeing Eden Energy Medicine practitioners, does not conduct live hearings with the kinds of procedures you would see in a court of law. Instead, the Ethics Committee ultimately makes its determinations based on the written record. Therefore, it is important that you document with precision the nature of your complaint and describe carefully the evidence you have for making the complaint. Describe what you have observed with specifics rather than providing only your interpretation of what the behaviors mean or imply.

4. The accused has the right to know who is making the accusation and the nature of the charge. For the Ethics Committee to open a case, the complaint must generally come from a party with direct knowledge of the alleged violation who is willing for the person who allegedly committed the violation to know who is making the charge. In your complaint, please give explicit permission that this information can be shared. Without it, a formal investigation of your complaint may not be initiated.

5. The Ethics Committee is obliged to respect the confidentiality of those involved. If you are naming individuals who are involved in the situation, but not being accused of an ethics violation, please indicate if the

Ethics Committee is authorized by you to inform them of how they are being mentioned and whether they know you have mentioned them.

6. The procedures to ensure due process are relatively complex and time-consuming. A ruling often takes at least three months from the initial complaint (in part because the Ethics Committee has to give people time to respond at various points along the way). In cases where there is concern of harm being done during this period, provisions exist for immediate temporary steps, but this is considered an extreme action.

7. The identity of the Ethics Committee members is not public knowledge, for a variety of reasons, but their identity is made known to the accused, who has the right to ask that any member of the committee who can be reasonably shown to hold bias be replaced by an alternative. An Innersource staff person will be assigned to carry out communications among the various parties.

8. Complaints should be submitted to ethics@innersource.net. Before submitting an ethics complaint, please also read the Eden Energy Medicine Ethics Committee "Overview and Procedures" (see appendix 3).

* * *

Points from the "Ethics Code for Energy Healing Practitioners" to consider prior to submitting an ethics complaint:

•   When EH practitioners believe there may have been an ethical violation by another EH practitioner, they attempt to resolve the issue by bringing it to the attention of that individual if an informal resolution appears possible and appropriate. Such interventions may not, however, violate any confidentiality rights that are involved.

•   If an apparent ethical violation has substantially harmed or is likely to substantially harm a person or organization and is not appropriate for informal resolution as described in the previous point, or is not adequately resolved in that fashion, EH practitioners take further action appropriate to the circumstances. Such action might include informing the appropriate ethics committee of the situation.

- EEM practitioners seek to promote accuracy, honesty, truthfulness, and dignity in the practice, teaching, science, and art of energy medicine.

- EEM practitioners do not falsely impugn the reputation of their colleagues, and do not file or encourage the filing of ethics complaints that are made with disregard for facts that would disprove the allegation.

Appendix C

Sample Ethics Committee Procedures

Following is the "Overview and Procedures" statements used by the Innersource Ethics Committee, which oversees Eden Energy Medicine (EEM) practitioners. It is provided here for our sister organizations to consider in developing their own ethics committee procedures and to inform readers of the *Ethics Handbook for Energy Healing Practitioners* about the functioning of health-care ethics committees.

Innersource Ethics Committee

OVERVIEW AND PROCEDURES

The Innersource Ethics Committee is established to review and act upon ethical complaints and concerns relating to the actions of:

- Innersource Certified Eden Energy Medicine (EEM) Practitioners
- Faculty and Students in the EEM Certification Program

For the purposes of this document, these individuals shall be collectively referred to as "practitioners." These practitioners have agreed in writing to stay informed of and to abide by the most current version of the "Ethics Code for Energy Healing Practitioners" posted at *www.EnergyMedicineEthics.com.*

The Ethics Committee shall be composed of three or more members, including Innersource's Board President as its Chair, or a person designated by the Board President to be its Chair, and a minimum of two EEM practitioners appointed by the Board President. Terms of office and number of Committee members beyond three are determined by the Board President. Committee meetings may be held in person, by telephone, or through the use of other electronic media at the discretion of the Committee Chair. The time and manner of Committee meetings are determined by the Committee Chair. Revisions to this "Overview and Procedures" document are made at the discretion of the Innersource Board of Directors.

Ethical conduct for EEM practitioners is defined by the most current posted version of the "Ethics Code for Energy Healing Practitioners" (see *www.EnergyMedicineEthics.com*) at the time of the ethical situation in question and as clarified and elaborated upon by the *Ethics Handbook for Energy Healing Practitioners.* Innersource reserves the right to take disciplinary action against practitioners, which may include but is not limited to the assignment of remedial education, reprimand, probation, suspension, and/or revocation of certification, or terminating a student from the Certification Program. Ethical complaints or allegations about an Innersource practitioner submitted to Innersource via e-mail, telephone, face-to-face meetings, letters, or through the Innersource website shall go to the Committee Chair. The Committee Chair may request that written complaints or allegations be clarified or that complaints or allegations delivered orally be submitted in writing before proceeding with an ethics review.

Before taking any action, the Committee Chair shall clarify issues of confidentiality. Professional standards of confidentiality and of informed consent shall be adhered to by the Committee in conducting its investigations. In general, if a person is presenting a complaint or allegation, that person must be willing to be identified to the person about whom the complaint or allegation is being made in order for an investigation to be initiated. If this agreement cannot be obtained, the matter may, at the Committee's discretion, lead to no further action. Instances in which no formal complaint or allegation has been submitted, but information of concern to the Committee comes via other channels, shall be adjudicated on an individual basis according to the best judgment of the Committee.

The Committee Chair is authorized to decide whether a complaint or allegation warrants attention by the entire Committee. If the Committee

Chair determines that (1) the matter is frivolous or inconsequential; (2) the complaint contains unreliable or insufficient information; or (3) the matter is not within the scope of Innersource's jurisdiction, then no further action will be taken and the complaint will be dismissed. In some instances, the Committee Chair or a person designated by the Committee Chair (this would generally be another Committee member or an Innersource professional staff member) has the right and sole discretion to bring about a resolution by facilitating communication among relevant parties, clarifying issues, or other direct actions. If this occurs, pertinent information will be included in a letter to the practitioner and the situation will be considered "resolved." The Committee Chair or designated individual also has the right and sole discretion to make alternative recommendations to the practitioner for resolving the issue before initiating a formal review.

After the Committee has opened a formal investigation, the Committee Chair or other designated individual shall send a letter to the practitioner informing him/her about the complaint, allegation, or situation (the "Complaint"). The letter can be sent via e-mail with receipt confirmed, or a letter sent by registered mail to the last address the practitioner provided to Innersource. The names of the Committee members shall be made known to the practitioner at that time. The practitioner has seven (7) days from receipt of notice of the names of the Committee members to submit in writing any objections to specific members of the Committee. Based on this or on information gathered from other sources, the Board President, in consultation with relevant parties, shall determine if specific Committee members should be recused to ensure a fair process, and if so, may appoint alternative Committee members for the case in question. Upon presentation of an ethical situation, Committee members are also asked to recuse themselves if they have a conflict that would compromise their ability to act objectively.

The practitioner has thirty (30) days from receipt of notice to submit a written response to the Complaint and/or present any additional evidence in support of his or her position. Failure by a practitioner to respond to the notice of a Complaint within the thirty (30) days shall be sufficient grounds to impose sanctions. Upon receiving a timely written request from a practitioner containing a reasonable explanation of the need for an extension, the Committee Chair may extend the period for the practitioner's response.

During the course of its investigation, the Committee may seek assistance or additional information from legal counsel, independent investigators, and any other appropriate individuals or organizations. All investigations are conducted objectively, with no prejudgment. Complaints will be considered without hearings, trial-type proceedings, witnesses, cross-examinations, appearance by practitioner, formal legal rules, or evidence and hearsay. Decisions by the Committee are based entirely on the written record. After receiving and reviewing the response from the practitioner, the Committee will review the available information and may take action or gather additional information before taking action.

If the Committee decides there is no violation of the Ethics Code, the Complaint is dismissed with written notice to the practitioner within fifteen (15) days of the completion of the investigation. If the Committee makes a determination that the Ethics Code was violated and imposes a sanction, the Committee will issue its decision in writing to the practitioner within fifteen (15) days of the completion of the investigation. Possible sanctions by the Committee include but are not limited to:

1. Decision of "no action" because of lack of grounds for action.
2. Decision leading to a formal reprimand from the organization.
3. Decision requiring retraining, remedial education, supervision, or professionally relevant personal development activities with specified mechanisms of updates to the Committee.
4. Decision to remove the individual from EEM practitioner lists, TA opportunities, or Innersource-sponsored teaching opportunities and to suspend use of Innersource professional credentials for a specified period of time.
5. Decision to remove the individual permanently from EEM practitioner lists, TA opportunities, or Innersource-sponsored teaching opportunities and to bar permanently the use of Innersource professional credentials.

If the practitioner is an EEM Certified Practitioner and the sanction imposed is suspension or revocation of certification, then the practitioner must cease from identifying or representing herself/himself as an Eden Energy Medicine practitioner. If the practitioner is a student in or faculty member of the EEM Certification Program, then the practitioner must cease from identifying or representing herself/himself as a student or faculty member, whichever is applicable.

An EEM Certified Practitioner, Certification Program student, or Certification Program faculty member and the subject of a Complaint may voluntarily surrender his or her certificate and/or status as a student or faculty member at any time before the Committee renders a final decision. Upon surrender, the Complaint will be dismissed without any further action by the Committee. In the event an EEM Certified Practitioner voluntarily surrenders his or her certificate, the practitioner must return his or her certificate to Innersource within thirty (30) days of notifying Innersource of such surrender and cease from identifying or representing herself/himself as an Eden Energy Medicine practitioner, faculty member, or student.

The Committee has the power to suspend the practitioner's Innersource activities and associations with Innersource while it is making its determinations, if it judges the Complaint to be of such a serious nature as to warrant this action.

The Committee's deliberations may be conducted privately at the Committee's discretion. The parties involved in a Committee action shall be informed of the Committee's conclusions within a reasonable period of time and at a level of detail determined by the Committee. If the Committee's action includes removing an individual from EEM practitioner lists, TA opportunities, or Innersource-sponsored teaching opportunities, or suspending or barring use of Innersource professional credentials, the Committee may inform Innersource staff and the practitioner's Innersource peers of this action as it deems appropriate.

Appendix D

Representing Yourself as an Energy Psychology Practitioner

Introduction

Energy psychology (EP) practitioners come from a spectrum of backgrounds, clinical orientations, and disciplines. Although all must navigate similar practice and ethical issues in bringing EP to the public, practitioners with different backgrounds and credentials must also operate within specific ethical, legal, and professional frameworks. This report offers a map of relevant issues for energy psychology practitioners according to their background and credentials.

EP practitioners fall into three practitioner categories in terms of licensure[7]:

1. **Licensed independent mental health professionals**. These individuals are trained and legally authorized to diagnose and treat mental disorders (as defined by the *DSM*).

---

7 All fifty states license conventional health-care professionals such as physicians, psychologists, nurses, social workers, and chiropractors. Other allied health-care professionals such as counselors, acupuncturists, massage therapists, and naturopaths are licensed in some states but not in others. State boards regulate the professional behavior of those within their jurisdiction, defining standards, ethics, and scope of practice.

2. **Other health-care professionals** whose license and training do not authorize them to diagnose or treat mental disorders.

3. **Unlicensed practitioners** encompassing a broad spectrum of disciplines, including life coaches, business consultants focusing on success in the workplace, and performance specialists working with athletes, singers, dancers, or actors.

Energy psychology clients, however, do not fit into neat categories. A businessman seeking help to be a better leader may be hindered by depression for which he is unwilling to see a mental health professional. A massage therapist may be working with a client who is, between sessions, emotionally traumatized during a robbery. An athlete's inability to reach her full potential may be limited by childhood messages from her parents. Your client's initial understanding of your scope of practice provides a foundation for you to be able to respond appropriately when such situations arise.

Five Basic Issues in Representing Your Energy Psychology Practice

In representing yourself to the public, several issues must be dealt with honestly and clearly in your advertising, website, informed consent procedures, and verbal statements. These include:

1. **Energy Psychology Is Considered an Experimental Treatment.**

   This concern applies most specifically to licensed independent mental health professionals, although any health-care practitioner utilizing energy psychology should consider it. Energy psychology for mental health issues is an alternative clinical approach that is controversial and not yet widely accepted within the conventional mental health community. It is not considered evidence-based or the "standard of care" at this time for any *DSM* disorder. This concern is usually addressed in informed consent forms.

   By no means, however, is it unethical to use an experimental approach, provided you have obtained proper informed consent. The public expects and has a right to a range of treatment options. It is certainly appropriate for you to describe your experiences and reasons for offering energy psychology methods and to present the theoretical basis and the growing body of evidence for the efficacy of the approach. The issue is *full disclosure* so your client can make an informed choice between a conventional approach and a less widely accepted approach. A legally sound informed consent and disclosure document is an essential risk management tool for your practice. In some cases, licensing boards or insurance providers may restrict the use of energy healing or other "experimental" practices, so it is, *as always,* essential to know the state and local laws and policies regulating the services you provide.

2. **People with *DSM* Diagnoses Will Contact You.**

This concern applies most specifically to unlicensed practitioners and health-care professionals whose license and training do not authorize them to diagnose or treat mental disorders. Even if you are not licensed to diagnose or treat *DSM* disorders, you are still likely to be confronted many times in your career with situations in which a person is coming to you for something other than a *DSM* disorder and, in the course of your intervention, the mental disorder may surface. Other times, the success of your work may involve helping clients overcome the impact of anxiety or depression or another *DSM* classification on their current life situation.

In some situations, you will easily recognize that the client's presenting problems are well beyond your training and that it is clear you need to make a referral and not attempt to address the *DSM* issue. However, because of the complexities and subtleties of human nature, it may not be at all clear-cut. Suppose you are the massage therapist mentioned earlier, providing weekly sessions to a woman who comes for preventive treatment after a history of back problems. You have taught her how to use energy psychology to better manage the stresses of daily life. You also use it occasionally during the sessions when emotional concerns arise that are interfering with the full effects of the massage treatments. One day, she comes in for her appointments obviously upset. She was the victim of an armed robbery three days earlier, and she finds herself shaking, ruminating about the event, and having nightmares, sleep difficulties, and other signs of the aftermath of a traumatic experience. She hopes you will use your energy technique to help her reduce her distress. Can you provide the treatment she is requesting for what is almost certainly a *DSM* disorder (technically, an "Acute Stress Reaction")?

The most fundamental guideline is that you cannot *diagnose* or *treat* a *DSM* disorder. You can, however, teach your client stress-reduction and relaxation techniques. That is within the scope of your license or training. If your intervention helps her to the point where she does not need further treatment, you have provided an appropriate service. If the intervention helps her, but not completely, or if the work on the recent trauma opens her to earlier traumas, you are at another decision-making point.

Having done what you can in the moment, a referral to a qualified mental health practitioner is probably called for. The gray line is—not being trained or licensed to make a diagnosis—how do you determine if it is probable that a *DSM* disorder is involved and referral to a mental health professional is required? This is a critical issue for people not licensed as mental health professionals who are nonetheless dealing with their clients' emotional issues. It is incumbent on you to receive the kinds of training that prepares you to make these determinations responsibly and for your client's highest good. Such training is available, and mental health professionals are also available for consultation in situations where you are unsure of the response that will best serve your client's welfare in a legal and professionally appropriate manner.

3.   **Be Clear, Accurate, and Descriptive About Your Credentials.**

This applies to all categories of practitioner. Anyone providing services to the public is required to represent relevant credentials (training, licensure, scope of practice) accurately, clearly, and in enough detail to avoid implications that are misleading. If you have a PhD, that is one of your credentials. If it is in chemistry, you need to specify this. The sources of your degrees, special certificates, and other relevant training should be made available to your clients in professional biographical statements on websites, brochures, or advertisements. Information about the nature of your license, including license number, should also be made easily available to the public. If a license, certificate, or diploma is not widely recognized or understood, such as the DCEP (Diplomate, Comprehensive Energy Psychology administered by ACEP, the Association for Comprehensive Energy Psychology), it should be explained.

4. **Be Clear if You Are Offering Two Different Sets of Services.**

   This concern applies most specifically to health-care professionals whose license and training do not authorize them to diagnose or treat mental disorders or to licensed mental health professionals whose licensing boards or insurance carriers use language that specifically disallows energy psychology or disallows experimental therapies. If you are a licensed health-care practitioner, such as a physician or massage therapist, who also offers energy psychology interventions for enhancing personal development, you are technically providing two sets of services. In most cases, the two sets of interventions will readily intermingle and complement one another. You must, however, be certain that you are working within your "scope of practice" as defined by your licensing board. This is particularly at issue if your energy psychology services are not primarily intended to supplement the health-care services you are licensed to provide, but are offered for goals independent of the scope of those services, such as enhancing professional performance, shifting self-defeating habits, or improving interpersonal relationships. At a minimum, your advertising and informed consent statements should ensure that your clients and prospective clients understand that you define the scope of your professional practice as incorporating an experimental modality. In some instances, it is necessary to operate separate practices for each service. This might involve discussing with the client when you are switching from one modality to the other (which must also be indicated in case notes and reflected in insurance billings if one modality is covered but not the other). At an extreme, some practitioners remove any chance for confusion or ambiguity by using separate offices, phone numbers, and advertising for providing each type of service.

5. **The Use of the Word "Psychology" in the Term "Energy Psychology" May Be Misleading.**

   This concern applies to all practitioners except licensed psychologists. The word "psychology" is used by historians, economists, politicians, behavioral scientists, and health-care practitioners who are not part of the profession of psychology. However, many states have strict regulations for the use of the terms "psychology" or "psychologist" or any of their derivatives in a manner that implies that one is practicing psychology. The practice of psychology may be defined in a variety of ways but almost always includes the diagnosis and treatment of *DSM* conditions.

If you are not licensed to diagnose and treat *DSM* conditions, *do not imply that you do!* Also, be very conscious of how you deal with the "gray line" discussed under point 2. In formulating public statements, advertising your practice, or promoting the field of energy psychology, you need to study the laws of your state and to seek the help of a qualified consultant or lawyer, if needed.

It takes little reflection to know that you cannot call yourself a psychologist if you are not one. Can you call yourself an "energy psychology practitioner?" This depends in part on your state laws, but it is ethically questionable, as it might imply that you have credentials in human psychology, psychopathology, and psychotherapy that you do not have and may make you legally vulnerable. Some states might even question the legitimacy of listing "Association for Comprehensive Energy Psychology" membership on your website, although such extreme interpretations of the restrictions on the use of the word "psychology" could probably be challenged legally.

Concluding Remarks

It is in your personal and professional interest, the interests of your clients, the interests of your community, and the interests of the profession that you represent your practice clearly and accurately and that you confine your practice to your scope of training and competence. Failure to comply with the laws and regulations that apply to you can result in substantial fines, lawsuits, and possible criminal prosecution. Whatever your level of training, licensed or not, it is also critical to create and maintain a referral network for clients you cannot serve effectively. If you have read this far, you are no doubt a practitioner who is committed to responsibly bringing more effective treatments to those who are suffering and more effective tools to those who wish to transcend their personal limitations and soar toward their peak potentials. We hope these guidelines will serve you in that intention.

References

Our two favorite ethics references could not be more different from one another. One is an easy and delightful read; the other a detailed 653-page text, including 671 case examples, which can serve like an ethics encyclopedia.

The Educated Heart: Professional Boundaries for Massage Therapists, Bodyworkers, and Movement Teachers, by Nina McIntosh, will speak to you in a highly personal manner and leave you immersed in the attitudes and principles of sound healing ethics. Quotations from *The Educated Heart* are placed throughout chapter 1 of this book, "Ethical Dilemmas You May Face."

Ethics in Psychology and the Mental Health Professions, by Gerald Koocher and Patricia Keith-Spiegel, while being directed toward the mental health professions, is unparalleled in its thorough treatment of the ethical issues that arise in all healing professions. It has been called by Kenneth Pope, one of the foremost leaders in professional ethics, the "gold standard" among ethics books that attempt to cover the entire vista of ethical issues. This is the book we consult when our organization is called upon to provide guidance on an ethics dilemma that is not covered by the *Ethics Handbook for Energy Healing Practitioners.*

The Toolkit for Energy Healing Practitioners includes forms, handouts, guidelines, business cards, brochures, and fliers that can be customized and printed, all designed for developing a successful energy healing practice. For more information about the *Toolkit,* visit *http://toolkit.innersource.net.*

Many other resources are also available. Among the most highly regarded books on health, medical, and psychological ethics are:

APA Ethics Code Commentary and Case Illustrations, by Linda Campbell et al. (American Psychological Association, 2010).

Clinical Ethics: A Practical Approach to Ethical Decisions in Clinical Medicine, by Albert R. Jonsen, Mark Siegler, and William J. Winslade (6th edition, McGraw-Hill Medical, 2006).

Creating Healthy Relationships: Professional Standards for Energy Therapy Practitioners, by Dorothea Hover-Kramer, MEd, RN (Energy Psychology Press, 2011).

The Educated Heart: Professional Boundaries for Massage Therapists, Bodyworkers, and Movement Teachers, by Nina McIntosh (2nd ed., Lippincott Williams & Wilkins, 2005).

Ethical Conflicts in Psychology, by Donald N. Bersoff (4th ed., American Psychological Association, 2008).

Ethics in Psychology and the Mental Health Professions: Standards and Cases, by Gerald P. Koocher and Patricia Keith-Spiegel (3rd ed., Oxford University Press, 2008).

Ethics in Psychotherapy and Counseling: A Practical Guide, by Kenneth S. Pope and Melba J. Vasquez (3rd ed., Jossey-Bass, 2007).

Ethics of Health Care: A Guide for Clinical Practice, by Raymond S. Edge and John Randall Groves (3rd ed., Thomson Delmar Learning, 2005).

Issues and Ethics in the Helping Professions, by Gerald Corey, Marianne Schneider Corey, and Patrick Callanan (7th ed., Brooks/Cole/Thomson Learning, 2007).

Practical Ethics for Students, Interns, and Residents: A Short Reference Manual, by Charles Junkerman and David Schiedermayer (University Publishing Group, 1998).

The primary text used in many energy healing classes is *Energy Medicine: Balancing Your Body's Energies for Optimal Health, Joy, and Vitality,* by Donna Eden with David Feinstein (rev. ed., Jeremy P. Tarcher/Penguin, 2008).

www.LearnEnergyMedicine.com

The Essential Guide for Building an Energy Medicine or Energy Psychology Practice

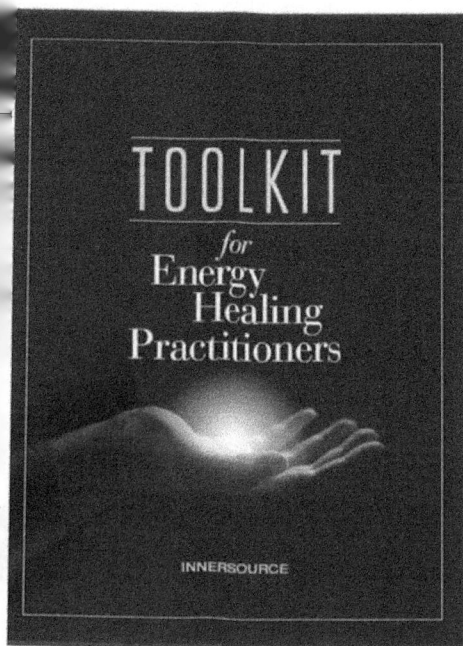

162 Separate Documents including:

- Checklist for starting a practice
- Intake, Referral, & many other forms
- Risk Management tips
- Client Handouts for back home practice
- When you must refer a client
- What to do if a client has a medical emergency during a session
- Press Releases and Web articles you can customize and use
- Detailed Informed Consent Statement
- Academic papers about EM & EP to send to skeptical colleagues
- Energy Medicine explained on a page
- Energy Psychology explained on a page

TOOLKIT
for
**Energy
Healing
Practitioners**

INNERSOURCE

Easy menu-driven navigation

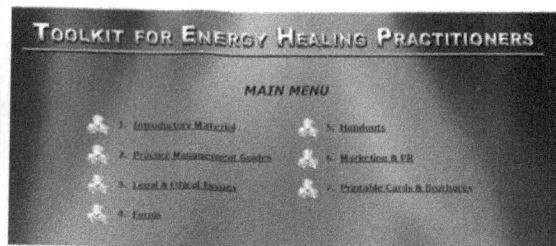

TOOLKIT FOR ENERGY HEALING PRACTITIONERS

MAIN MENU

1. Introductory Material
2. Practice Management Guides
3. Legal & Ethical Issues
4. Forms

5. Handouts
6. Marketing & PR
7. Printable Cards & Brochures

$159 Retail
Publisher's Discount $129
http://toolkit.innersource.net
800-835-8332 (24 hour order line)
541-488-7662 (questions and/or orders)

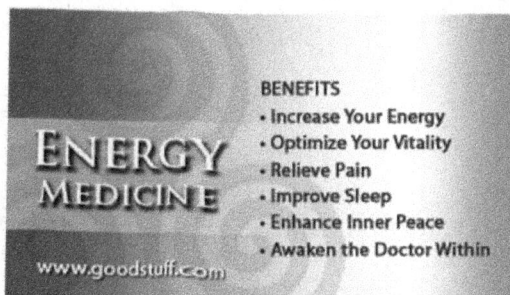

BENEFITS
- Increase Your Energy
- Optimize Your Vitality
- Relieve Pain
- Improve Sleep
- Enhance Inner Peace
- Awaken the Doctor Within

**ENERGY
MEDICINE**

www.goodstuff.com

Back of one business card format
See full-color samples at
http://toolkit.innersource.net

90 versions of business cards, fliers, and brochures you can customize and have printed and mailed to you.